Medicine and Public Health Through Time

For AQA GC

Acknowledgements

The front cover shows 'The Stone of Madness' by Brueghel, The Bridgeman Art Library.

The publishers would like to thank the following individuals, institutions and companies for permission to reproduce copyright illustrations in this book:
AKG London 8, 42, 64, 78; AKG London/Erich Lessing (Paris, Musée du Louvre) 24, 27, 40; Alfred Pasieka/Science Photo Library 162; Atlantic Syndication Partners 157; Bettmann/Corbis 91, 122 (top),131; Bibliotheque Nationale de France 58; Bodleian Library 60, 79; Bond McIndoe Centre, Queen Victoria Hosptial 148, 136 (top left); Bridgeman Art Library 56, 101; Bridgeman Art Library (Cheltenham Art Gallery) 96; British Library 66 (Cotton Augustus AVI F66), 67 (Slo 6F1 77v), 68 (Harl 3729 ff158v-159), 69 (ADD 47680 f 54V), 71 (Slo 1977 f 6V), 82 (Henricus Martelus), 97 (Jacob Rueff), 103 (History of London by W Maitland); British museum 18, 19; Canterbury Museums 52; Chris Hellier/Corbis 39; Collection of Musée de l'Homme 9; Corbis 136 (bottom left & top right), 143 (right), 159 (left), 160; Crown Copyright 156, 136 (bottom right); Araldo de Luca/Corbis page 22; Directorate of Education and Culture, Museum of South Yorkshire Life, Doncaster 141 (left); Direktion der Museen der Stadt Wien 74; Dr Jeremy Burgess/'Science Photo Library 125; E D Hoppé/Corbis 10; Ecole Nationale Supérieure des Beaux-Arts, Paris 28; Eigentum des Germanischen National Museums 65; English Heritage Photo Library 38; English Heritage Photo Library/Jeremy Richards 46, 48; English Heritage Photo Library/Jonathan Bailey 49; Foto Roncaglia 61; Frognal Centre, Queen Mary's Hospital, Sidcup, Kent 147 (bottom left & right); Guildhall Library 93; Holt Studios International 159 (top); Hulton Deutsch 114;Hulton Deutsch/Corbis 136 (top right); Hulton Getty 106, 111, 122 (bottom), 140, 141(right), 150, 151, 152; Imperial War Museum 147 (top); Jean-Loup Charmet/Science Photo Library 128 (top); Life File 47, 159 (centre); Mary Evans Picture Library 119, 129, 133 (right); Mauro Fermariello/Science Photo Library 154, 136 (bottom centre); Metropolitan Museum of Art, gift of Ernest and Beata M. Brummer, in memory of Joseph Brummer, 1948, 35; Michael Nicholson/Corbis 86; Moredun Scientific Ltd/Science Photo Library 123 (right); Museo Vaticano/Scala 32; National Medical Slide Bank 153; National Monuments Record, English Heritage 95; National Portrait Gallery, London 115; Österreichische Nationalbibliothek 62; PA Photos 159 (right); Photo RMN-Hervé Lewandowski, Louvre 16, 17, 22; Public Record Office Image Library 92; Punch Publications 110, 116; Roger Woods/Corbis 15; Royal Collection Enterprises 83; Royal College of Physicians 90; Russell Kightley Media 161; Scala 36; Science Museum/Science & Society Picture Library 128 (bottom); Science Photo Library 143 (left); Sir William Dunn School of Pathology, University of Oxford 144; Sonia Halliday Photographs 73; Su Davies/Life File 20; Masters and Fellows of Trinity College, Cambridge 72; Wellcome Library, London 43, 44, 63, 70, 76, 84, 85, 87, 88, 89, 94, 109, 123 (left), 124, 133 (left), 155.

The publishers would also like to thank the following for permission to reproduce material in this book:

American College of Physicians for an extract from Annals of Internal Medicine by Barquet and Domingo, 1997; HarperCollins Publishers Ltd for an extract from The Greatest Benefit to Mankind by Ray Porter, 1997; Joseph Henry Press, Washington DC for an extract from The People's Health by Robin Marantz Henig, 1996; Longman for an extract from Medieval England – Towns, Commerce and Crafts by Edward Miller and John Hatcher, 1995; Oxford University Press for an extract from Growing up in Medieval London: The Experience of Childhood in History by Barbara Hanawalt, 1995; Palgrave for an extract from History of Medicine: A Scandalously Short Introduction by Jacalyn Duffin, 2000; Random House Group for an extract from The Medieval Town by Colin Platt, published by Martin Secker & Warburg.

Every effort has been made to trace and acknowledge ownership of copyright. The publishers will be glad to make suitable arrangements with any copyright holders whom it has not been possible to contact.

Orders: please contact Bookpoint Ltd, 130 Milton Park, Abingdon, Oxon OX14 4SB. Telephone: (44) 01235 827720, Fax: (44) 01235 400454. Lines are open from 9.00 – 6.00, Monday to Saturday, with a 24 hour message answering service. Email address: orders@bookpoint.co.uk

British Library Cataloguing in Publication Data

A catalogue record for this title is available from The British Library

ISBN 0 340 80112 3

First published 2002

Impression number	10 9 8 7 6 5 4 3 2 1
Year	2008 2007 2006 2005 2004 2003 2002

Typeset by Liz Rowe.

Printed in Great Britain for Hodder & Stoughton Educational, a division of Hodder Headline Plc, 338 Euston Road, London NW1 3BH by Printer Trento.

Medicine and Public Health Through Time

For AQA GCSE Specification A

Tony McAleavy, Derek Patterson
and Martyn Whittock
Editors: David Aldred and J.A. Cloake

Hodder & Stoughton
A MEMBER OF THE HODDER HEADLINE GROUP

Contents

Welcome to Prehistory

Timeline

2.5 million BC	First stone tools used by early humans
150,000 BC	First modern humans evolve
10,000 BC	Humans have migrated to every continent in the world except Antarctica
8,000 BC	First farming takes place – change from Old Stone Age to New Stone Age

What was prehistoric medicine?

In this book you will find out about medicine through time, starting with the medicine of the prehistoric people who lived thousands of years ago. 'Prehistoric' means before the invention of writing. The discovery of writing not only changed how people lived, it also created new sources that we can use to make sense of the past. We know very little for certain about medicine before the invention of writing. In the absence of written sources much of our evidence comes from the findings of **archaeologists**.

Hunter-gatherers

Prehistoric people lived as 'hunter-gatherers'. They hunted wild animals and gathered the nuts, vegetables and fruits that grew naturally. Modern men and women belong to a biological group known as *homo sapiens*. The first examples of *homo sapiens* are known from about 150,000 BC. In 10,000 BC there may have been about 5 million people in the whole world. This is fewer than live in one large city, like London, today. These Stone Age men and women were not necessarily worse off than the people who came later. One of the themes that will run through your study of the history of medicine is the idea that progress is not inevitable and does not follow a simple line through time. In many ways life got worse for people when they stopped being hunter-gatherers and became farmers.

What do we know about the world of the Stone Age?

Our knowledge is limited by the evidence. Without any writing we depend on archaeological findings, such as:

- skeleton remains and burial sites

- findings from caves that were used as shelters or religious sites.

Using evidence of this kind we can work out some of the features of Stone Age life.

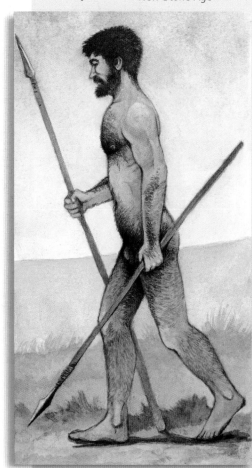

▲ SOURCE A Archaeologists have excavated the bones of prehistoric men and women at a place called Cro-Magnon in France. This reconstruction shows a Cro-Magnon man.

KEY WORD

archaeologist – a scientist who tries to find out about the past by looking at objects left behind by people in the past

QUESTION

Look at some of the educated guesses we can make about Stone Age people:

- Hunters were nomads: they wandered from place to place in search of food. They travelled across **land** that was largely empty of other people. An area the size of Britain would only contain a few thousand people. The hunters travelled in small tribal groups or 'bands' of about 40 people.

- They had no permanent **homes** but lived in temporary shelters or caves. Human waste was easily got rid of and people moved on before much dirt and waste had built up.

- There was no **government** and no one, outside the hunting band, to turn to if things went wrong.

- **Food:** Meat was usually plentiful because there were so many wild animals and so few people. The meat of wild animals is usually of a very good quality. Stone Age people could make fires and used fire for cooking. However, the cooking was not always successful and sometimes half-raw meat was eaten. For vegetables, people gathered edible wild leaves, roots and berries. People knew a lot about these different plants.

- There was lots of clean **water** available from streams and rivers.

- The nomadic hunting lifestyle provided lots of **exercise** for people.

Using this information would the following aspects of Stone Age life have made people more or less healthy? Complete the table below with the information from the bullet points.

Aspect of Stone Age Life	More healthy	Less Healthy
Land		
Homes		
Government		
Food		
Water		
Exercise		

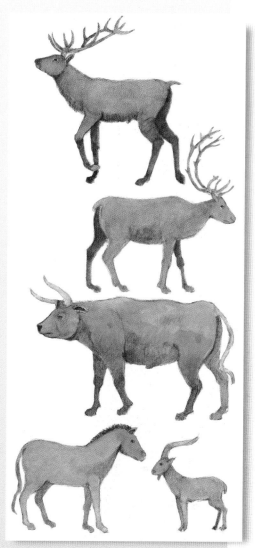

▲ SOURCE B The excavations at Cro-Magnon have shown that prehistoric men and women at this site hunted and ate: reindeer, red deer, aurochs, horse and ibex.

enquiry

What can we learn about prehistoric medicine from archaeological evidence?

Look at the following archaeological evidence about prehistoric people. Try to work out what each piece of evidence tells us about prehisto medicine.

Evidence One: Human Bones

Human bones can last a very long time and tell us a lot about health and how long people lived. The bones of Stone Age people show that few men survived over the age of forty, and women often died younger still. Archaeologists can tell that the painful bone disease arthritis was often common among Stone Age people.

In many parts of the world, archaeologists have come across a very strange phenomenon. They have discovered circular holes in the skulls of Stone Age people. We know that Stone Age people had sharp stone tools and it seems that they used these tools to make these holes. We can also tell from the way the bone has grown that these mysterious holes were often made while people were alive. This must have been both very painful and very dangerous. Scientists use the word trephination to describe the operation of cutting a hole in the skull. Why would people agree to this painful, dangerous operation? Was trephination a form of prehistoric medicine?

▲ SOURCE A Archaeologists can tell that this operation took place while the person was alive. We also know that the patient survived. How might we tell?

KEY WORD

trephination – a surgical operation in which a circular piece of bone is removed from the skull; sometimes also known as *trepanation*

☑ EXAM TIP

Make sure that you understand the problem of archaeological evidence in relation to our knowledge of early medicine.

Evidence Two: Cave paintings

Archaeologists have found many beautiful cave paintings made by prehistoric people, especially in caves in modern France and Spain. Many paintings show the animals that these people hunted. Some paintings seem to show people carrying out ceremonies or rituals.

In one famous painting from France, a man is shown wearing the antlers of a stag. He is dancing. The cave with this painting is known as 'The Three Brothers'. Who is the Stag Man of the Cave of the Three Brothers? Can you think of any possible links between this painting and medicine in prehistoric times?

◄ SOURCE C The strange figure painted on the walls of The Three Brothers Cave in France. It seems to show a man dressed as a stag.

▼ SOURCE B Roberto Margotta writing in 1967. One Italian historian thinks there are strong links between our two pieces of evidence and prehistoric medicine. Let's look at his views:

In one cave in France, The Three Brothers, a rock engraving has been found which dates back 17,000–20,000 years. It shows a doctor wearing a monstrous deer-mask over his face. He is the typical sorcerer of a primitive community. Animal masks like this were worn to frighten away the demons causing the illness and to impress the patient, so that he would be impressed by the sorcerer's spells and rituals. They made spells to make people sick and spells to make people well. Sorcerers were also the first to practise trephining. The place where the cutting took place suggests that surgery was for specific purposes, such as relieving headache or epilepsy. It is also possible that the sorcerer wanted to remove a tormenting demon from the skull.

QUESTIONS

1   What was trephination?

2   What does the cave painting of The Three Brothers' Cave show?

3   Explain in your own words how Roberto Margotta interprets the prehistoric bones and cave paintings.

4   Margotta seems very sure about his interpretation of the evidence. Do you think he is right to be so sure about prehistoric medicine? In your answer you should refer to each piece of evidence and mention:

   • what we can *tell for certain* from the two pieces of evidence

   • what we can *only guess* from the two pieces of evidence

   • in conclusion what we can learn about prehistoric medicine from archaeological evidence.

enquiry

Can Aboriginal ideas help us find out about prehistoric medicine?

In the last unit we saw how an Italian historian used archaeological evidence to find out about prehistoric medicine. He said that:

- prehistoric people believed that illness was caused by spirits

- there were special sorcerers who used magic to make people better.

▲ **SOURCE D** Australian Aborigines until very recently lived a hunter-gatherer lifestyle similar to prehistoric men and women. What can we learn about prehistoric medicine by studying the Aborigines?

How can we check whether Roberto Margotta was right? There is a limit to what we can be sure about when looking at faint traces of archaeological evidence. One way of trying to find out more about prehistoric medicine is by looking at the lifestyle of a more recent hunter-gatherer people.

The Aborigines of Australia are one such people. Until Europeans reached Australia in the late eighteenth century, the Aborigines lived as hunter-gatherers, without farming and without writing. If similar conditions lead to similar ideas we may be able to learn about prehistoric medicine by studying Aborigine medicine.

Aborigines travelled about in search of animals to hunt and wild vegetation. Their homes were temporary shelters. They had no writing but they were great story-tellers and artists; this artistic tradition continues today. Their nomadic lifestyle kept them fit and allowed them to leave dirt and waste behind them when they moved on. They travelled in small groups and had contact with few other people, and this reduced the chance of contracting infectious diseases.

Aborigines used magic to treat disease. They believed that spirits caused disease in different ways. Evil spirits, they thought, sometimes entered people and made them sick. The good spirits that lived inside people sometimes left, and this too caused illness. Sometimes spirits entered or left because of witchcraft. Aborigines believed that it was possible to deliberately use spells to make an evil spirit invade the body of an enemy. This was done with the help of a special bone, known as a pointing bone. These pointing bones could also be used to remove a good spirit from the body of an enemy.

Some Aborigine people specialised in curing people by the use of magic to drive out evil spirits. These are sometimes known as 'medicine men' or 'clever men'. This is a little misleading because in some tribes there were also women who practised magical cures. The medicine men treated patients by chanting repetitively, sending a patient into a trance and massaging the sick parts of the body. If the problem was an invasion of the body by an evil spirit, they called upon the spirit to leave the body. Sometimes they announced that they had removed the evil spirit and trapped it in a quartz crystal. Treatment was different if a spirit had been taken from a patient's body by witchcraft. The medicine men then had to find the pointing bone, and release the missing spirit by throwing the bone into water.

The Aborigine people were skilled at looking at the natural world and had many practical skills. As hunters and gatherers they needed these skills to survive. They relied on wild vegetation for food and they acquired practical knowledge about the healing qualities of many of these plants. They could treat **dysentery**, for example, by chewing the bulb of an orchid. They were able to treat simple wounds and fractures. Broken arms were placed in clay and allowed to heal. Open cuts were 'bandaged', with such materials as bark or kangaroo skin, until they had healed. The sap of bracken was used to ease the pain from insect bites. Some of these practical Aborigine treatments are now widely used beyond Australia. One example is the use of Tea Tree leaves. Aborigines burnt the leaves to make a vapour that was good for breathing problems. Today people in many different parts of the world use the oil of the Tea Tree leaf as a treatment for cold symptoms.

QUESTIONS

1 Using archaeological evidence, Roberto Margotta came to the following conclusions about prehistoric 'medicine':

- Spirits were believed to be a cause of disease.

- They had special ceremonies and treatments to deal with spirits.

- They had sorcerers or magicians with supernatural powers.

For each of the points explain whether his views are supported by the evidence from Australian Aborigines.

2 What additional information about medicine can we gain from the Aborigine evidence?

3 Why do historians use aborigine evidence to find out about prehistoric medicine?

KEY WORD

dysentery – a painful and dangerous disease of the intestines, which involves severe diarrhoea

☑ EXAM TIP

Make sure that you understand that prehistoric and Aboriginal medicine was based upon *supernatural* thinking, but there are problems of evidence. Remember that there is clear evidence that people carried out surgery.

Welcome to the Ancient Civilisations: A Change for the Better?

About ten thousand years ago a great revolution took place in the Middle East. People learned to grow crops and keep animals, instead of hunting them. They began to give up the life of wandering and settled down in permanent settlements. The age of farming had begun, and with it a new way of life that we call 'civilisation'. Slowly the new lifestyle spread to other parts of the world. This great change in the way people lived had a big impact on health and medicine. But were the changes all for the better? Look at these six consequences of the introduction of farming. For each one decide whether it is evidence of *progress* or *regress*. These are important ideas in your study of medicine: progress is change for the better, regress is change that makes things worse.

Farming produced more food than hunting so the human population began to rise. Nomadic hunter-gatherers probably had no choice but to abandon very sick or elderly relatives who could not keep up with the rest. No longer forced to move constantly, sick and very old people could now be looked after.

The development of diseases such as **malaria** was closely liked to the arrival of agriculture. Malaria was caused by a parasite carried by the mosquito, and mosquitoes thrived in agricultural land carved out of the wilderness.

Archaeology shows that the first farmers were often less well-fed than their hunter-gatherer ancestors. This is indicated by the fact that skeletons of the Old Stone Age are, on average, taller than the New Stone Age skeletons of the first farmers. The farming families ate a narrow range of starchy foods, such as bread. This provided enough calories for survival but contained a limited range of vitamins and other nutrients.

KEY WORD

malaria – a feverish disease, spread by mosquitoes; the symptoms can come back again and again

Life in farming villages provided many opportunities for disease to spread. Houses were often dirtier than the temporary camps of hunters. People could no longer move on and leave their waste behind them. As villages grew and the first cities emerged, people came into contact with larger numbers of other, disease-bearing humans.

The first farmers kept large herds of cattle and these were a source of new human disease. Many of the diseases that have caused great human suffering started as cattle diseases, and crossed over to nearby human populations.

Farming eventually led to another revolution: the development of writing. Farmers needed to keep a tally of their work, stores and harvests. About 5,000 years ago people in the Middle East learned to how to write on soft clay, using pens made from reeds. The development of writing made possible records of new scientific discoveries.

overview
Welcome to Ancient Egypt

Timeline

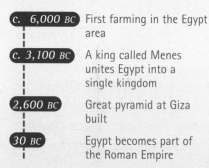

c. 6,000 BC First farming in the Egypt area

c. 3,100 BC A king called Menes unites Egypt into a single kingdom

2,600 BC Great pyramid at Giza built

30 BC Egypt becomes part of the Roman Empire

In about 3,000 BC a powerful state emerged in Egypt. The Egyptians were remarkable builders and the most famous symbols of their civilisation are the huge pyramids of Giza, built around 2,600 BC. Many of the ancient Egyptians were farmers. Their lives were dominated by the great River Nile that flowed through the farmlands of Egypt. Every year the Nile flooded and the flood waters were used to irrigate the land. Egyptians were ruled over by a very efficient government that grew rich by taxing the farmers. At the head of the government was the king, known as the Pharaoh. This man had great power and was seen as a god on earth. The Egyptians were skilled at writing. They used a form of picture writing known as hieroglyphics. They wrote on clay tablets and on a form of paper made from a reed called papyrus.

The Egyptians were good at many practical things but they were also religious and superstitious. They could quarry huge amounts of stone for their buildings. They knew how to construct artificial channels to water their fields. Despite this practical side to their culture they often turned to religion to explain mysterious events. They believed that life was controlled by a group of powerful gods. Many of these gods were a mix of human and animal characteristics. Egyptians believed that crops only grew because of the god Osiris and his wife, Isis. Osiris had to die and be re-born each year in order to help the crops. They believed that there was a powerful sun god called Re or Ra, who journeyed across the sky each day in a boat. There was a good and bad side to most of the Egyptian gods; depending on their mood they could help or harm people in their everyday life. The Pharaoh was central to their religion. By performing the correct ceremonies he had the power to please the gods and stop them from causing harm.

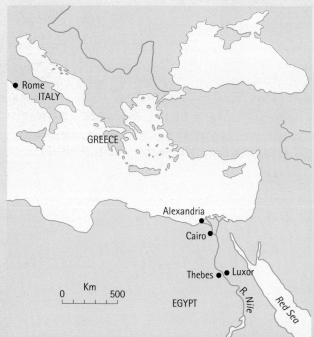

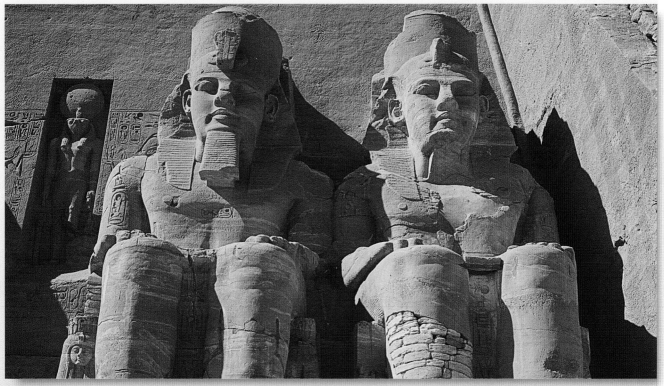

▲ **SOURCE A** These enormous statues of the Pharaoh Ramesses II give some idea of the great power of the rulers of Egypt. What does the picture tell us about the skills or capabilities of the people who built them?

QUESTIONS

1 Think about the information on this page. Can you see any clues that explain why there was important medical progress in the Egyptian period?

2 Source A shows a picture of a series of giant statues of an Egyptian king. What can we learn about the Egyptians from archaeological evidence like this?

3 Can you see any clues that explain why Egyptians used both natural and supernatural approaches to disease? Put the information in a table like the following one:

Belief in practical approaches to problems	Belief in supernatural approaches to problems

enquiry

How did the Ancient Egyptians change medicine?

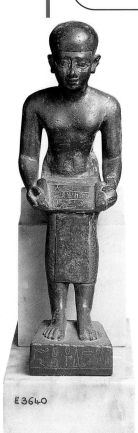

E3640

▲ **SOURCE A**
Imhotep was doctor to a pharaoh called Djoser. After his death Imhotep was worshipped as a god of medicine.

When we considered prehistoric medicine we had difficulty finding out what life was like in the past because there were few sources of information to help us. We know a lot more about Egyptian medicine because there are many more sources of information:

- There are many inscriptions that tell us about doctors and medicine.
- Eight medical books have survived written on papyrus.
- The bodies of wealthy Egyptians were embalmed (preserved using chemicals) and many have survived. Scientists can learn about typical medical problems by studying these bodies.
- Towards the end of the Ancient Egyptian period several Greek writers visited Egypt and described Egyptian life, including medicine.

The practice of medicine is so divided among them that each physician treats one disease, and no more. There are plenty of physicians everywhere in Egypt. Some are eye-doctors, some deal with the head, others with the teeth or the belly, and some with hidden maladies …

▲ **SOURCE B** A Greek visitor, Herodotus, who visited Egypt in the fifth century BC. He was surprised and impressed by the way doctors specialised in different parts of the body.

Who were the first professional healers?

In Ancient Egypt there were, perhaps for the first time in history, many full-time doctors. In a wealthy society, people could pay full-time specialists to treat them. Some of these doctors were also priests. There were female doctors and healers. One woman, called Peseshet, is described on a carving as the head female physician. One of the earliest known Egyptian doctors was called Imhotep, who lived about 2,700 BC. As well as being a doctor, he was an adviser to the Pharoah Djoser. Many centuries after his death the Egyptians began to worship him as a god of healing.

Today there are doctors who are 'general practitioners' and doctors who are 'specialists'. The general practitioners are family doctors with a wide knowledge of common medical problems. The specialists are experts in just one area of medicine. There was a similar development in Ancient Egypt. Specialist healers treated specific parts of the body. There were, for example, dentists as well as eye doctors.

☑ EXAM TIP

Remember the significance of the introduction of writing – it both helped doctors of the time to learn treatments and gives historians evidence of people's thinking about medicine in Ancient Egypt.

Doctors and religion

One important group of priest-doctors particularly worshipped the goddess, Sekhmet. She was feared as a powerful goddess who could send either sickness or cures depending on her mood. Other doctors included followers of the god Thoth. In one medical papyrus it says, 'The good doctor is guided by Thoth. The god's knowledge is found in scrolls that are read by the wise.'

As this source suggests, doctors relied heavily on the way medicine was carried out in the past, as recorded in old writing. There were medical books of guidance that they were expected to follow. A Greek visitor noticed this and the fact that failure to follow the written instructions could lead to severe punishment.

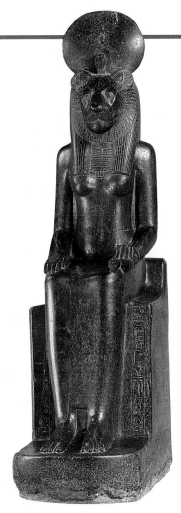

▲ **SOURCE D** Sekhmet: a goddess with the body of a woman and the head of a lion. Egyptians believed that, depending on her mood, she had the power to cure or to cause illness.

If they follow the rules of this law as they read them in the sacred book and yet are unable to save their patient, they are absolved from any charge [they won't be put on trial]; but if they go contrary to [against] the book's teachings they must submit to a trial with death as the penalty.

▲ **SOURCE C** Diodorus, a Greek writer and historian of the first century BC.

Successful Egyptian doctors were often very well paid. The tomb of a doctor called Nebamun shows a man and a woman being handed medicine. In return they have a line of servants ready to hand over a lavish fee. The payment includes several slave girls. The richest and most powerful doctors worked for the ruler of Egypt, the Pharaoh. We know that one royal doctor called Iry was also the high priest. A tomb inscription describes him as 'the king's eye doctor', 'doctor to the king's belly' and 'guardian of the king's anus'! The last title refers to his responsibility to provide the Pharaoh with drugs that would empty the bowels.

QUESTIONS

1   Why do we know much more about medicine in Ancient Egypt than prehistoric medicine?

2   What medical help could you get if you were a rich Egyptian?

3   Compare the information about doctors in Ancient Egypt, with the information about Aborigine medicine men on page 11. What differences are there in the way the two societies provided medical care? Can you see any similarities between the two societies? You could comment on their ideas about illness, the job of healers and how they passed on medical knowledge.

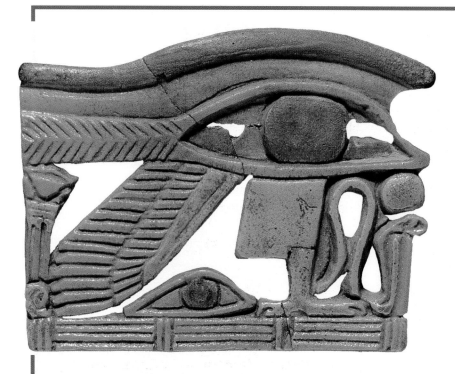

What anatomical knowledge did the Egyptians have?

Anatomy is an important aspect of medicine; it refers to knowledge about the inside of the human body. The surviving papyrus documents show that the Egyptians had a good idea of the key internal parts of the body, including the heart and the lungs. They also understood some of the ways in which these parts of the body were connected together. Egyptian doctors saw the heart as the key. The heart was where both the soul of a person was to be found and thinking took place. The heart was connected to the rest of the body by channels called 'metu'. The channels carried air and blood and many other fluids: tears, saliva, urine, faeces, sperm. The 'metu' also carried bad substances called 'wehedu' that caused illness.

2 Explain what Egyptians meant by 'metu' and 'wehedu'.

It is sometimes said that Egyptians learned about how the body worked through mummification. Most modern historians reject this idea. They believe that embalming added little to Egyptian medical knowledge. Embalmers worked in secret. They were a completely different group from the healers and there is no evidence that there was much contact between them. Embalmers removed organs through the nose and through small slits in the body so as to do as little damage as possible to the body. They avoided altogether opening bodies up in a way that would have increased anatomical knowledge. Egyptian doctors probably learned more from the way animal bodies were cut for ritual sacrifice.

The secret knowledge of the heart and the heart's movements:
46 channels go from the heart to every part of the body. If a doctor, a priest of Sekhmet or a magician, places his hand on the head, hands, stomach, arms or feet then he hears the heart. The heart speaks out of every limb. There are four channels in the nose, 2 for mucus, 2 for blood. There are four channels in the forehead which give blood to the eyes ...

▲ SOURCE F An account of the inside of the body from one of the surviving Egyptian medical books the *Ebirs Papyrus*.

3 What can we learn from Source F about Egyptian knowledge of anatomy?

How did the Egyptians explain and treat disease?

Egyptians believed that people could become sick for both natural and supernatural reasons. Evil spirits could enter the body and make a person sick. People could also become ill if they displeased a god. Alternatively, the body's channels could become clogged up with 'wehedu': rotten food and faeces. People could avoid illness by pleasing the gods and keeping the body's channels clear of any blockages. Once a person had fallen sick remedies were either religious or practical.

4 Look at the following extracts from the medical papyri. For each one decide whether it is evidence of a supernatural or a natural explanation of disease.

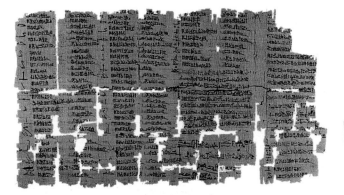

▲ **SOURCE G** This papyrus document has survived for over 3000 years. Papyrus texts provide a mass of information about Egyptian medical beliefs.

A cure for burns

Mix milk of a woman who has born a male child with gum and ram's hair. While putting the mixture on the burn say the words of the Goddess Isis, 'My son, Horus is burnt in the desert. Is there any water there? There is no water. I have water in my mouth and a Nile between my thighs. I have come to extinguish the fire.'

A diseased wound in a patient's chest

Examine a diseased wound in the chest and inflammation of the wound. The man continues to be feverish from it.
Make cool applications to draw out the inflammation from the mouth of the wound.
Apply leaves of willow and dung.
Make an application to dry up the wound.
Apply green powder, salt and grease.

A wound in the head

Feel the wound to make sure that the skull is not injured.
You should bind fresh meat upon it on the first day and cover it with two strips of linen. On later days apply grease, honey and lint every day until he recovers.

KEY WORD

diagnosis – finding out the type of medical problem that someone suffers from by observing their symptoms

A cure for cataracts

Mix brain of tortoise with honey. Place on the eye and say 'There is shouting in the southern sky in darkness. There is an uproar in the northern sky. The crew of the Sun God, Ra bend their oars. Ra will drive away the God of Fevers.

Concluding your enquiry:

How did the Egyptians change medicine?
- List prehistoric ideas and methods
- List Egyptian ideas and methods
- Identify key changes (i.e. the move from supernatural to natural cures).

overview

Welcome to Ancient Greece

Timeline

c. 800 BC Small city states emerge in Greece

800–600 BC Greek settlers establish Greek colonies throughout the eastern Mediterranean

500–400 BC Greek civilisation reaches its peak

338 BC Greek city states are conquered by Philip, king of Macedonia

Many important changes took place in Greece between 500 and 350 BC. To make sense of these changes we need to know about some key features of life in Ancient Greece.

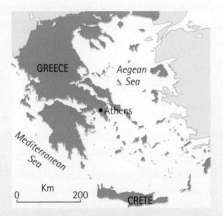

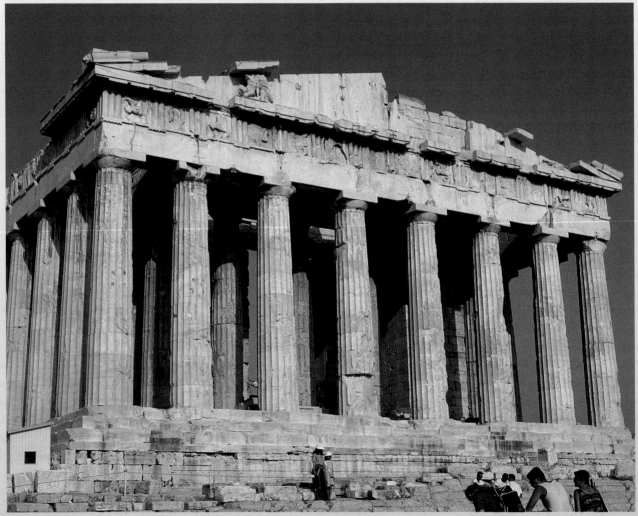

▲ **SOURCE A** The temple of the Parthenon in Athens is often seen as a symbol of the achievements of the people of Ancient Greece.

RELIGION

Greek religion was based on belief in a number of powerful gods, who lived on a mountain in heaven called Olympus. The most important God was Zeus. In the 6th century BC some Greeks began to attack the idea of the gods of Olympus. Increasingly, some educated Greek people stopped taking the gods seriously. They said that the stories about the gods could not be literally true. Belief in the gods did not disappear; some educated and many uneducated people continued to worship the old gods.

EDUCATION

In most Greek states education was thought to be important. It was expected that all male citizens would be able to read and write. Many developed a great love for books and ideas. The Greeks also valued physical education. They believed that a healthy fit human body was a thing of great beauty. Greek men took part enthusiastically in athletics competitions.

WHO WERE THE GREEKS?

GOVERNMENT

Although all Greeks shared the same language and many traditions, they did not belong to one state and they were not ruled over by one government. Instead the Greeks were organised into many small city states. Sometimes big powerful governments try to control what people say and think. This was not possible in Ancient Greece. People were free to develop new ideas. If they did not like the government of their local city state, they could always move to another Greek state.

SCIENCE

Some Greek men were passionately interested in making sense of the world. They were called 'philosophers': in Greek this means 'lovers of wisdom'. They rejected the idea that you could explain what happened in nature as the result of the actions of the gods. Instead, they looked for scientific reasons.

☑ EXAM TIP

Make sure you can work how each of these key features could encourage people to discover new medical knowledge.

enquiry

Why was Asklepios important in Greek medicine?

The Asklepion

The world of Ancient Greece was complex. Long before Hippocratic doctors, there were religious healers. Many people worshipped a healing god called Asklepios (sometimes spelt the Roman way Asclepius). The work of the Hippocratic doctors (explained on pages 24–7) did not lead to a decline among followers of Askelpios. Worship of Asklepios seems to have increased during the years when the Hippocratic books were being written. An Asklepion, a temple to Asklepios, was set up in almost every known city in the Ancient Greek world. Over 200 such temples are known. Sick worshippers spent time at the temple and hoped for a cure. The greatest Asklepion was at a place called Epidauros.

It seems that some people in Ancient Greece clung on to their beliefs in the gods. Others tried Hippocratic medicine first, were sometimes disappointed by the results and then turned to the god Asklepios. Asklepion medicine was free; Hippocratic doctors charged for treatment. In Source B, one poet from Athens described how he had tried to get a cure from Asklepios only after ordinary doctors had failed:

> *Despairing of human skill but with all hope in the divine,*
> *Leaving Athens, blessed in her sons, and coming to your grove,*
> *Asklepios, I was cured in three months of a wound*
> *In the head that had lasted for a whole year.*

▲ SOURCE B From a poem by the Greek poet, Aischines.

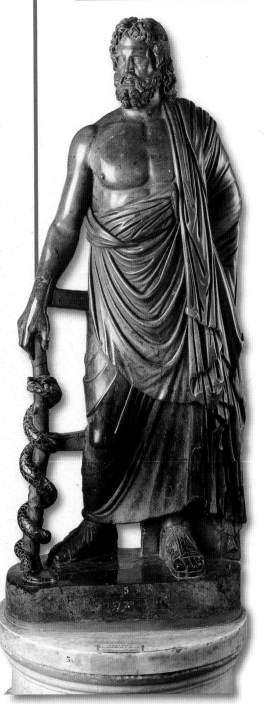

▲ SOURCE A A Statue of Asklepios, the god of healing. A snake wrapped around a staff was the symbol for Asklepios and is still used today as a symbol for healing.

When archaeologists dug at the site of the Asklepion at Epidauros they found a staggering 10 cubic metres of offerings to the god in the shape of parts of the human body. These offerings depicted every imaginable part of the body including: arms, legs, hands, eyes, breasts and genitalia. Source C below shows people making offerings to Asklepios.

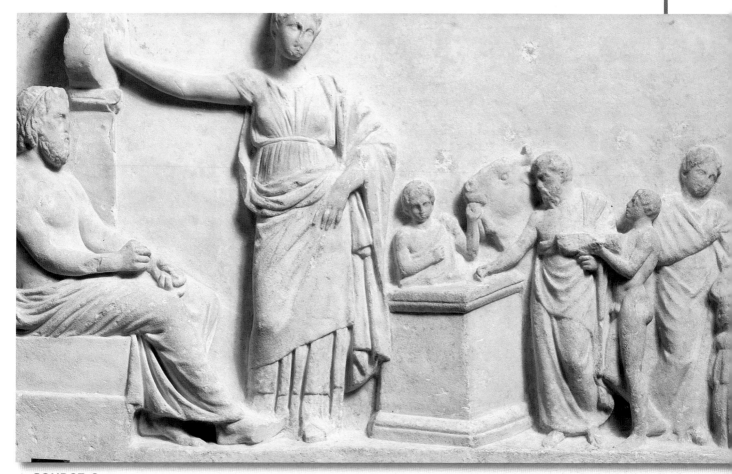

▲ **SOURCE C** This carving shows the seated figure of the god Asklepios and his daughter Hygieia. The smaller figures sacrificing a bull to Asklepios for good health.

QUESTION

Describe what happened at the Asklepion.

enquiry

How important were Hippocratic ideas?

The most important changes that took place in Greek medicine were linked to the name of a doctor called Hippocrates. We know very little about the real Hippocrates. According to tradition he was born on the island of Kos in about 460 BC and he spent much of his life working on the island as a doctor. He died in about 380 BC. There is a collection of 60 medical books supposedly written by Hippocrates, known as the Hippocratic Collection. Hippocrates cannot have written all these books because they were written at different times between 430 and 300 BC. It is clear that many different people wrote these books – so we can learn little from Hippocrates about how individuals changed the course of medicine. Despite this, Hippocrates is significant because the people who called themselves Hippocratic doctors had a new approach to medicine. Hippocratic medicine was based on a number of key ideas:

Clinical observation
Hippocratic doctors were very careful about the way they looked at patients and recorded their symptoms. These methods are known as 'clinical observation' and are similar to the way doctors work today. The Hippocratic doctors kept detailed 'case notes', recording how the illness developed. By building up lots of case notes they were able to predict how an illness would develop. These ideas are summed up in two Greek words that are still used by doctors today:
- *'diagnosis' – the cause of a disease was identified by a careful consideration of symptoms*
- *'prognosis – the outcome of the disease was predicted.*

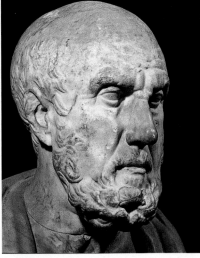

▲ SOURCE A Hippocrates. We know very little about this Greek doctor but his followers changed the nature of medicine.

A rejection of supernatural explanations
The Hippocratic doctors insisted that you could not explain disease by talking about supernatural forces. They also rejected the idea that you could make yourself better by ritual cures, such as spells and cleansing ceremonies. There were many magicians and priests who offered such treatments. The Hippocratic doctors saw these as rivals and tricksters.

Regimen: the importance of diet and exercise

*While ready to use blood letting, vomiting and purging, Hippocratic doctors also believed in **preventive medicine**. The best way of making sure that the humours stayed in balance was through exercise and diet. The Hippocratic doctors talked about 'regimen': healthy lifestyle.*

KEY WORD

preventive medicine –   taking action to avoid illness

The Four Humours: A new theory of disease

The followers of Hippocrates believed that there were four fluids or 'humours' in the human body: blood, phlegm, yellow bile and black bile (see page 22). Different humours increased at different times of the year. Illness occurred when there was too much of a particular humour. The Hippocratic doctors talked about the need for a balance of the humours to keep a body healthy. They thought that the body naturally tried to get rid of excess humours: that was why the nose produced mucus during a cold. Doctors could help the body to balance the humours by blood-letting, by vomiting and emptying of the bowels.

Ethical behaviour

Hippocratic doctors believed that being a doctor was a very special job. Responsibilities were spelt out in a solemn promise made by new doctors known as the Hippocratic Oath. This stated that doctors would never mistreat their patients.

QUESTIONS

1   Explain the following aspects of Hippocratic medicine in your own words:

   - rejection of magic

   - clinical observation

   - the Four Humours

   - preventive medicine

   - the Hippocratic Oath.

2   Identify the aspects that built on Egyptian ideas and those which were new. Which do you think were more important?

3   Why did Asklepion medicine remain popular long after Hippocratic methods were introduced?

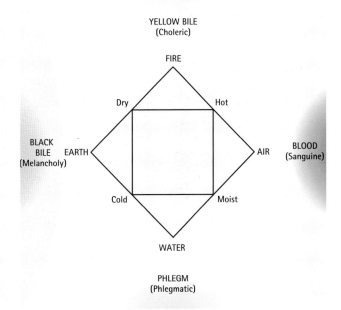

▲ SOURCE B The four humours and the four basic elements.

Examples of Hippocratic writings

QUESTIONS

1   Look at the following extracts from Hippocratic writings. Each source provides evidence for at least one of the key ideas of Hippocratic medicine. For each source work out a link with a key idea.

2   Which of the sources is most useful for a historian finding out about explanations of disease?

3   Which of the sources is most useful for a historian finding out about what Greek doctors did?

I do not believe that epilepsy is a 'sacred' disease. People who think it is caused by the gods view it with ignorance and superstition. Those who first called this disease 'sacred' were quacks and charlatans. By talking about the gods they hide their own ignorance and their inability to give suitable treatment.

▲ SOURCE B

At Meliboea, a young man who had a temperature for a long time as the result of too much drink and too much sex, took to his bed. His symptoms were shivering, nausea, insomnia and lack of thirst.
First day. His bowels passed a large quantity of solid faeces accompanied by much fluid.
Following days. He passed a large quantity watery, greenish stools. His urine was thin and small in quantity, and of bad colour. He took deep breaths at long intervals. His upper body was swollen. Palpitation of the heart. He passed oily urine.
Twentieth day. Went mad, much tossing about, passed no urine, kept down a small amount of fluid.
Twenty Fourth day. Died.

▲ SOURCE A

Run and wrestle during the winter. In summer, wrestling should be restricted and running forbidden, but long walks in the cool part of the day should take their place.

▲ SOURCE D

I will use my power to help the sick to the best of my ability. I will harm no one with my medical knowledge. Whenever I go into a house, I will go to help the sick and never with the intention of doing harm or injury. I will not abuse my position to obtain sex with women or men, free or slave.

▲ SOURCE C

Vomiting should be encouraged during the winter months, as this is the time when phlegm dominates and diseases are to be found in the head and the chest. The emetic [a medicine to make you vomit] should consist of ground hyssop in six pints of water, drunk after adding vinegar and salt. During the summer enema [medicine to empty the bowels] should be used as this is the hot season when the body is more bilious.

▲ SOURCE E

☑ EXAM TIP

The usefulness of sources depends on their relevance to a topic, so your answers to questions 2 and 3 will be different.

Biography

Aristotle: A Great Greek Thinker

One of the greatest scientists of Ancient Greece was Aristotle (384–322 BC). Aristotle was the son of a doctor, and among other jobs he worked as tutor to Alexander the Great, who was a great military leader. As well as his contribution to medicine, Aristotle wrote about an astonishing range of subjects: politics, philosophy, ethics and astronomy.

Aristotle is important in the history of medicine because of his work developing biology: the study of living things. Aristotle said that all biology – including medicine – should be based on a methodical observation of plants and animals in the real world. His belief was that there was always a purpose to everything that Nature did. He carried out dissections of animals – but not humans – to find out how they worked.

Aristotle made a special study of how young creatures grew. He saw the heart as the key organ of the body. He studied the connection between blood vessels and the heart, although he did not understand the difference between **arteries** and **veins**. Aristotle saw the heart as the place where body heat was produced. By contrast he saw the brain as a kind of refrigerator that cooled down the body. The heat of the body was regulated by these two organs working together.

Aristotle had an influence on scientists for many centuries. In the Middle Ages his writings were held in great respect. His influence continued into the Renaissance period and beyond. William Harvey, who in the seventeenth century discovered how the heart caused blood to circulate around the body, was a great admirer of Aristotle and based his own scientific method on the work of the Greek scientist.

QUESTION

Aristotle was not a doctor. Does this make him unimportant in the history of medicine? In your answer mention:

- whether people other than doctors can increase medical knowledge

- how Aristotle increased medical knowledge.

KEY WORDS

artery – a blood vessel that carries blood away from the heart

vein – a blood vessel that carries blood back to the heart

enquiry

Why was Alexandria important in Greek medicine?

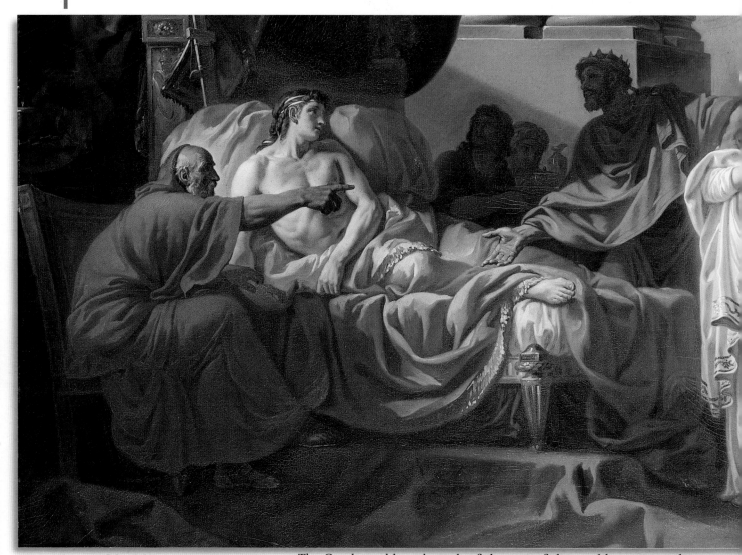

▲ **SOURCE A** An eighteenth-century painting showing Erasistratos diagnosing the love sickness of Antiochus, the king's son. Erasistratos dissected the human body and identified features of the brain.

The Greek world, and much of the rest of the world, was turned upside down by the amazing conquests of an extraordinary leader known to history as Alexander the Great. He founded a great new city in northern Egypt, known as Alexandria, in 331 BC. Although this city was in Egypt, it was part of the Greek cultural world and its richest people spoke and wrote in Greek. After the death of Alexander, Egypt was ruled by the Greek family of one of his soldiers, a man called Ptolemy. These rulers developed Alexandria as a great centre for writers and scientists. In the third century BC Alexandria was the most important centre for the study of medicine in the world. Its most famous medical researchers were called Herophilos and Erasistratos.

KEY WORDS

cerebrum – the front part of the brain

cerebellum – the back part of the brain

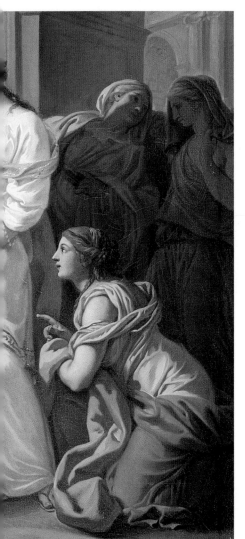

Herophilos increased understanding of the pulse. He established the importance of measuring the pulse as part of clinical observation. Herophilos also understood that there was a link between the pulse and the beat of the heart.

Erasistratos studied anatomy and, in particular, the workings of the human brain. He worked out that all nerves were linked to the brain. He identified distinct parts of the brain, such as the **cerebrum** and the **cerebellum**. Erasistratos criticised earlier ideas that nerves were filled with air. He established, instead, that they were solid.

These discoveries were only possible because dissection was permitted in Alexandria. Herophilos dissected dead bodies at public exhibitions. This had not been possible earlier in Greek history. It was also said that Erasistratos experimented on live human beings, possibly condemned criminals.

Alexandria was eventually taken over by the Romans and became part of the Roman Empire. It remained an important medical school until the last days of the Roman Empire.

QUESTIONS

1 How did medicine at Alexandria differ from earlier Hippocratic medicine?

2 Why are Herophilos and Erasistratos important in the history of medicine?

☑ EXAM TIP

The best answers to questions that ask 'how important was', are the ones that make comparisons between different things.

Concluding your enquiry:

Why was Alexandria important in Greek medicine?
• Re-read your answers to this enquiry

• Write down why the Asklepion was important

• Write down why Alexandria was important

• Explain which you think was more important.

overview

Welcome to Rome and its Empire

Timeline

510 BC	The Roman Republic was set up
300–100 BC	Rome conquers most of the territory around the Mediterranean
31 BC	First emperor, Augustus takes power
400–500 AD	Roman power in western Europe declines

Who were the Ancient Romans?

Between 300 and 100 BC a powerful new state began to dominate the world of the Mediterranean. It was centred on the Italian city of Rome. The power of Rome continued to spread. The Greek mainland was under Roman control by 146 BC. By the first century AD the Romans ruled over much of Europe, north Africa and the Middle East. A ruler called Augustus took power in 31 BC and became the first emperor of Rome. Roman emperors continued to rule over their enormous sprawling empire for the following four centuries.

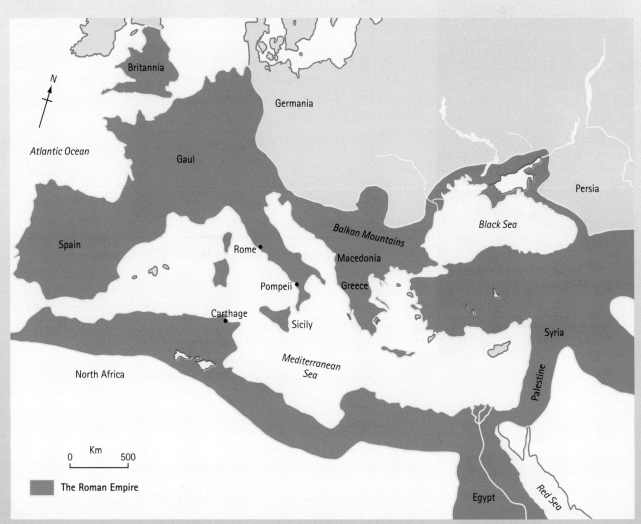

▲ **SOURCE A** The Roman Empire in AD117.

The Romans had a very powerful and **well-organised government**. As different people were conquered they were forced to pay taxes that contributed to the wealth of the Roman government. Local wealthy people were usually recruited to the side of the Romans and ruled provinces on behalf of Rome.

The ability of the Roman government to rule over so many different people depended on the strength of **the Roman army**. In its heyday the Roman soldiers were able to defeat almost any other army. They were very disciplined and well organised. They also had good equipment. Roman soldiers were not only good at fighting. They built magnificent roads so that they could march quickly to any trouble spots.

Religion remained a powerful force in the Roman world. Traditional Roman religion was very similar to Greek religion; they believed that there were gods and goddesses who controlled the lives and fortunes of people. The Romans were very tolerant of different religious ideas and allowed many different religions and cults to thrive and spread. Towards the end of the Roman Empire the Christian faith spread and finally became the official religion of the Empire.

Romans were not very original thinkers. The Romans had **a 'love-hate' relationship with the Greeks**. They took many ideas from the Greeks and Greeks influenced much Roman thinking about such things as architecture and science. At the same time many rich Romans looked down on the Greeks because they were not tough enough and were too interested in books and ideas. The Romans liked to see themselves as much more practical and down-to-earth than the Greeks.

☑ **EXAM TIP**

In the exam you shoud show how different aspects of a society, such as Rome, had an important impact on medical knowledge. Look at the information on this page and make sure that you can work out how each of these key features might affect medicine.

enquiry

What did the Romans learn from the Greeks about medicine?

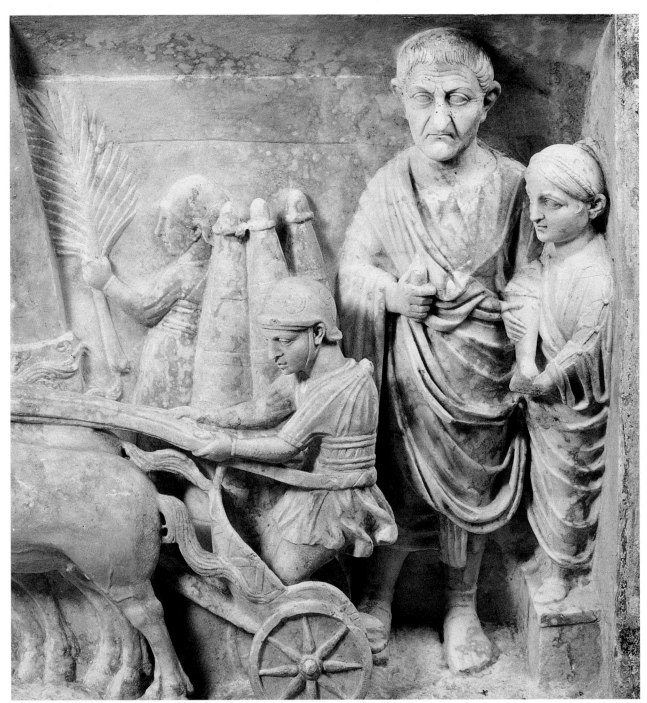

▲ **SOURCE A** A carving showing a Roman man and his wife. Roman husbands were very powerful and they traditionally looked after medical matters for their family.

Roman medicine before contact with Greece

In many ways medicine in the early days of Rome was much more primitive than Greek or earlier Egyptian practice. There were, at first, no full-time doctors in Rome. Instead families were expected to take care of their own medical problems. Family medicine was male-dominated. The father of the family took the lead and was taught medical remedies by his own father. This traditional Roman family medicine was very simple. The early Romans were farmers who put much trust in the healing powers of a small number of farmyard materials. In particular, they were great believers in the healing power of wool and cabbage. Unwashed new wool was mixed with animal fat and the herb rue. This mixture was used on cuts, bruises and swellings. Women were given rams' wool mixed with oil to relieve inflammations. Wool mixed with oil was also used for back pains. Romans believed that cabbage had many health-giving properties and that the urine of someone who had eaten cabbage was good medicine. As farmers, the first Roman writers on medicine saw little difference between the treatment of farm animals and humans.

All matters relating to the health of men and cattle can be taken care of without the services of a physician, and all illnesses can be treated by the chief herdsman.

▲ **SOURCE B** Varro, a Roman writer who specialised in agriculture and lived in the first century BC.

If you have reason to fear sickness, give the patient or the oxen the following before they get sick: 3 grains of salt, 3 laurel leaves, 3 leek leaves, 3 spikes of leek, 3 of garlic, 3 grains of incense, 3 plants of Sabine herb, 3 leaves of rue, 3 stalks of bryony, 3 white beans and 3 pints of wine. You must gather, mash, and administer all these things while standing and he who administers the remedy must be fasting. Administer the medicine to each ox or patient for three days.

The urine of a person who has been living on a cabbage diet should be kept as medicine. When warmed up this urine is a good remedy for diseases of the muscles. If you wash little children with this urine, they will never be weak and puny.

▲ **SOURCE C** Cato, a Roman politician and writer who lived 234–149 BC.

QUESTIONS

1 Describe how medical care was provided in the early days of Roman history.

2 'Early Roman medicine was primitive compared to Hippocratic medicine.' Do you agree with this statement?

enquiry

Why did the Romans resist the arrival of new doctors from Greece?

From about 200 BC full-time Greek doctors began to appear in Rome and other parts of the Roman world. We have seen that the Romans had a fairly simple sense of medicine and had no full-time doctors before this. Surprisingly, the new, well-educated Greek doctors were greeted with hostility by many Romans. Can you think of any reasons why a change like this would be opposed? Look at the following statement by a Roman writer; what does it tell use about the Roman approach to doctors?

> *Our ancestors did not condemn healing but they disapproved of medicine as a job. They did not like the idea of making money from saving lives. Of all the Greek sciences, only medicine has not yet gained wide interest among us sober and serious-minded Romans.*
>
> *Any man off the streets can call himself a doctor. We trust these doctors because of our desperate hope of being healed. We ought to have laws against the ignorance of doctors. They risk our lives while they are learning. Their experiments lead to deaths, and yet for doctors, and only doctors, there is no penalty for killing a man. In fact, they pass on the blame, criticising the dead themselves for their lack of moderation and self-indulgence.*

▲ SOURCE D Pliny the Elder, a Roman military leader and writer. He was killed when Mount Vesuvius erupted in AD79.

Despite the views of people like Pliny, Greek doctors continued to make the journey from Greece to Rome. Eventually Greek doctors became an accepted part of the society of the Roman Empire. These doctors were followers of the Hippocratic tradition and gave their advice based on belief in the Four Humours.

What part did religion play in Roman medicine?

The Romans not only made use of Greek doctors but also looked to the religious approach to healing developed by other people in Greece. The Romans liked taking the gods of different people and making them part of their own religion. Many Romans liked the cult of Asklepios. They changed his name to Aesculapius and built a temple to this Greek healing god right in the centre of the city of Rome. The idea of the Asklepion even reached Britain. Near Lydney, in the Forest of Dean, the Romans developed a healing centre that seems to have been run on the same lines as an Asklepion. At Lydney the healing god was a local god called Nodens; people stayed the night and hoped that the god would visit them and bring a supernatural cure.

☑ EXAM TIP

Exam questions sometimes ask why new ideas in medicine were opposed by people. Use this enquiry as an example of this.

▶ SOURCE E
A Greek doctor in Rome. He is reading a medical text and he has medical instruments on top of his cupboard. Many Romans were suspicious of doctors like this.

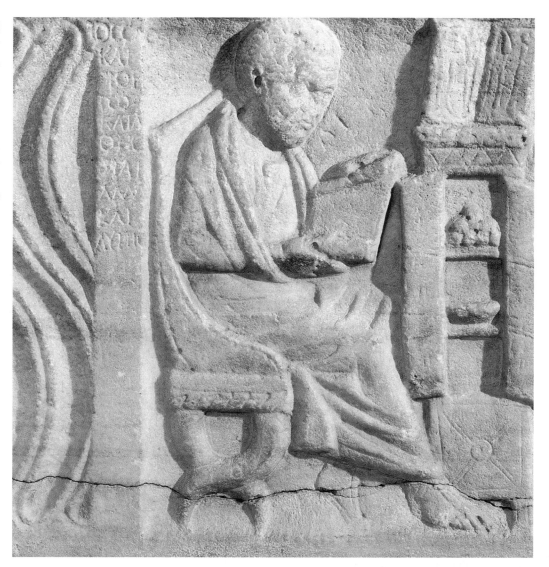

QUESTIONS

1 Using Source D and your background knowledge explain why there was hostility towards Greek doctors when they moved to Rome.

2 How do we know that the Romans were interested in Greek religious ideas about healing?

enquiry

Medicine and the common people: What was the Roman approach to public health?

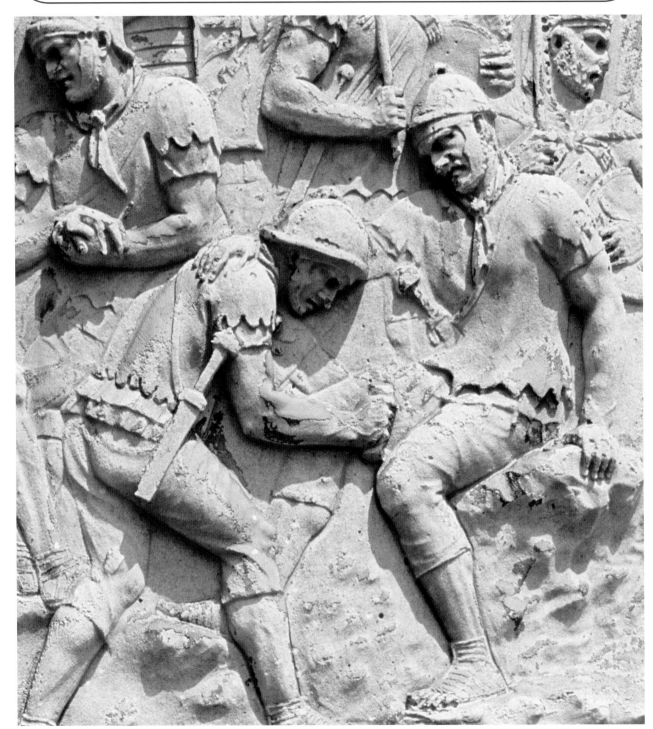

▲ **SOURCE A** A wounded Roman soldier is helped on the battlefield. The Roman army had medical specialists called 'medici'.

How did the Romans look after the health of their army?

The Roman army was, in its heyday, extremely well organised and effective. The medical care of ordinary soldiers was taken very seriously. The treatment of the wounded was very well organised. Some soldiers were trained both to fight and to look after the wounded. These specialists were known as '*medici*'. They were not doctors but they did have enough basic medical training to cope with battlefield emergencies. We can see the 'medici' at work on a very famous carving in Rome known as Trajan's Column. This carving of the first century AD shows fighting between Romans and their enemies in the area of modern Hungary.

Away from the battlefield the Roman army also had special hospitals to care for the sick and the wounded. These were known as '*valetudinaria*'. The hospitals were built to an identical regular plan all across the empire. One of these hospitals has been excavated by archaeologists at Inchtuthil in Scotland. It had wards separated by spacious corridors and an elaborate system of drains and sewers.

Through experience the Romans understood that **epidemic diseases** could spread quickly and disastrously among an army. The steps they took to stop illness among the army give us insights into Roman views of medicine.

> **KEY WORD**
>
> epidemic disease – a disease that spreads rapidly and affects many people

> *I will now give you some ideas about how the army can be kept healthy, by the siting of camps, purity of water, temperature, exercise and medicine. Soldiers must not remain for too long near unhealthy marshes. A soldier who must face the cold without proper clothing is not in a state to march. He must not drink swamp water. The generals believe that daily exercise is better for soldiers than going to see doctors. If a group of soldiers is allowed to stay in one place for too long then they begin to suffer from the effects of polluted water, and are made miserable by the smell of their own excrement. The air becomes unhealthy and they catch diseases. This has to be put right by moving to another camp.*

▲ **SOURCE B** Vegetius, a Roman who wrote about the army in the fourth century AD.

QUESTION

Describe how a Roman soldier was kept fit for fighting.

enquiry

Planning settlements

The Romans believed that some places were healthier than others. They took great care to put any new town, farm or army camp in a place that they thought would be healthy. Look at these descriptions of good places for settlement. What can we learn from them about Roman ideas about the causes of disease?

A marshy neighbourhood should be avoided. For when the morning breezes blow towards the town at sunrise, they bring with them mists from the marshes and, mingled with the mist, the poisonous breath of the creatures of the marshes which wafts into the bodies of the inhabitants. This will make the site unhealthy.

▲ **SOURCE A**
Vitruvius, a Roman writer on architecture of the first century BC.

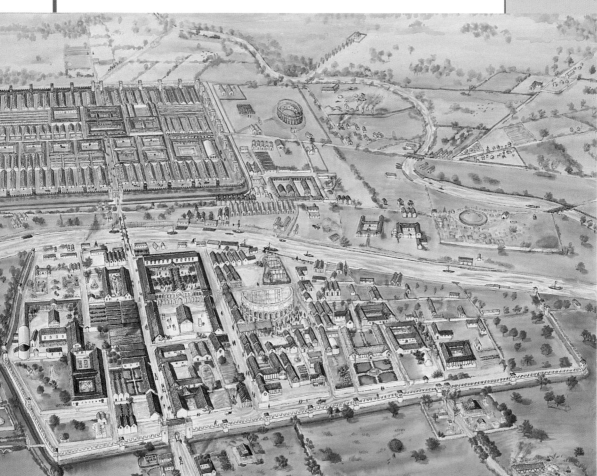

▲ **SOURCE B** A reconstruction drawing showing Roman York in AD209. The city has two parts: a legionary fortress on one side of the river, and a civilian settlement on the other side. The Romans took great care when locating settlements like this.

When building a house or farm special care should be taken to place it at the foot of a wooded hill, where it is exposed to health-giving winds. Care should be taken when there are swamps in the neighbourhood, because certain tiny creatures which cannot be seen by the eyes breed there. These float through the air and enter the body through the mouth and nose and cause serious diseases.

▲ **SOURCE C** Varro, a Roman writer on agriculture of the first century BC.

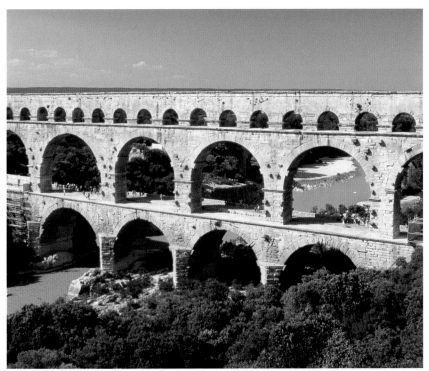

▲ **SOURCE D** In some parts of the Roman Empire bridges carrying Roman aqueducts can still be seen today. This aqueduct is near Nimes in southern France.

The new Anio aqueduct takes water from the river which is muddy and discoloured because of the ploughed fields on either side of the river. Because of this a special filter tank was placed at the beginning of the aqueduct where the soil could settle and the water become clear before going along the channel. Six other aqueducts have similar filter tanks outside the city.

▲ **SOURCE E** Frontinus.

The water supply

The Romans believed in the importance of clean water to health. They used great ingenuity and technical skill when finding ways of transporting water to their cities. Water was carried in large pipes or conduits (open channels) made of brick or stone. These structures were called aqueducts. In some places extraordinary bridges were built to carry the pipes across valleys. Some of these were so well constructed that they still stand today. Most aqueducts were not bridges; the pipes ran on or underground.

One Roman writer, called Frontinus, was in charge of the water supply for Rome itself at the end of the first century AD. (This was a very important and prestigious job; Frontinus also had other important jobs during his lifetime, including being Governor of all Britain). Frontinus saw the water supply as essential for the existence of the city. 'My office ... concerns not only the usefulness of such a system, but also the very health and safety of Rome ...'. He compared the great practical achievement of Roman public health to the 'useless' pyramids, and the clever, but impractical ideas of the Greeks.

As the capital city, Rome had a very elaborate water supply system. At the time of Frontinus Rome was served by nine long-distance aqueducts. Four of these came from the Anio Valley in the hills above Rome. The water of the Anio was described by the Roman writer, Pliny as, 'The most famous in the whole world for coldness and wholesomeness'. Great effort was involved in building and maintaining the aqueducts, and they ran over great distances. The new Anio Aqueduct, for example, was 87 kilometres long. Thousands of workers were needed to build such structures, and Frontinus had a team of hundreds of slaves to help him keep them in good working order.

The aqueducts of Rome delivered a remarkable amount of water to the city. At the time of Frontinus the daily delivery was 173 million litres a day. Most of this went to public bath-houses, street fountains and government buildings. Private houses were not usually connected to the system. Most families had to collect water by hand from one of the public fountains. Very rich people could pay a special charge and get piped water.

enquiry

The baths

One of the reasons why Roman government took such great efforts to get good water supplies was because of their belief in the benefits of bathing. Public baths were a key feature of life in Rome and most Roman towns. Both men and women used the baths on a regular basis; some people went once a day. Some baths were free, others made a small charge. They usually offered a range of baths of different temperatures, as well as areas for gymnastics and other sports. Going to the baths was an important social event. People could buy food and gossip with their friends at the baths.

Public lavatories and sewers

In addition to the baths, the Roman authorities also provided public lavatories in most Roman towns. In the city of Rome there were 150 public lavatories in the fourth century AD. There was little privacy in these places. Like the baths, lavatories were places where people met and gossiped. Instead of toilet paper the Romans used a sponge on a stick. These were provided in public lavatories. They were rinsed after use and then re-used. One Roman writer described how an unhappy gladiator committed suicide by ramming a lavatory sponge down his own throat. Larger Roman towns had sewers to carry away human waste from the public lavatories.

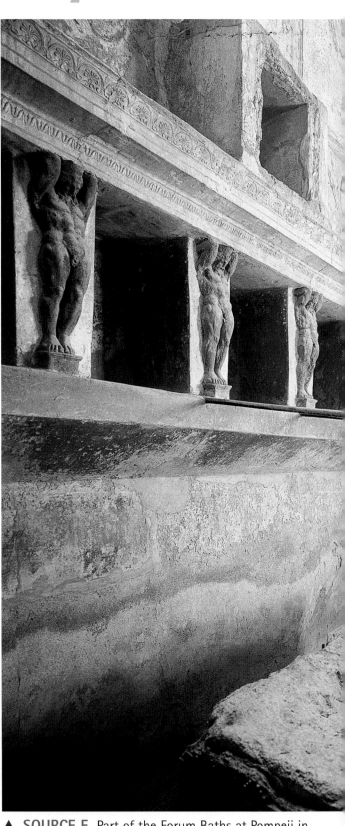

▲ **SOURCE F** Part of the Forum Baths at Pompeii in Italy. Public baths like this were an important feature of cities across the Roman Empire.

Old men still admire the city sewers, the greatest achievement of all. They were built 700 years ago. There are seven rivers made to flow in seven tunnels under the city, these finally run into one great sewer. These rivers rush through like mountain streams and, swollen by the rain water, they sweep away all the sewage. The bottoms and the sides of the sewers take a real hammering.

▲ **SOURCE E** Pliny the Elder, first century AD.

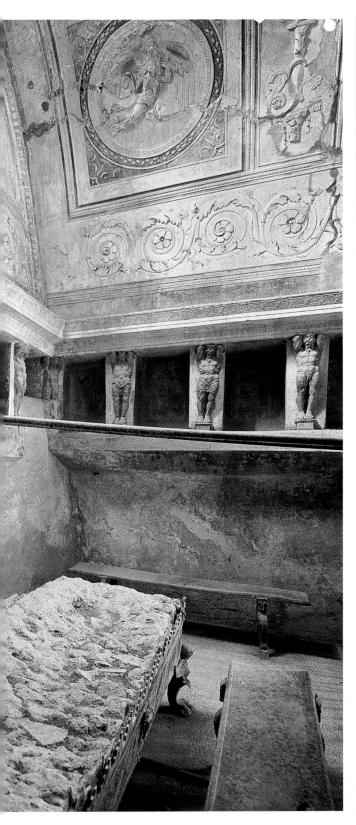

I have next to speak of those who have some weak part of the body. Such a man should go to the baths. He should first stay wrapped up and sweat in the tepidarium *[warm room]. Then he should be anointed with oil. Next he should go to the* caldarium *[hot room]. After a further sweat he should not go as usual into the hot bath but should have a shower from the head downwards, first with hot, then tepid, and finally cold water. This should be poured longest on the head. Nothing is so good for the head as cold water.*

▲ **SOURCE G** Celsus, a Roman medical writer of the first century AD.

QUESTIONS

1 What was the Roman approach to Public Health? Write a detailed answer that draws upon information from throughout this unit. In your answer you should describe:

 - the location of camps and settlements

 - the supply of clean water

 - public baths

 - sewers and sanitation.

2 Look at each aspect of Roman Public Health you have described. What ideas about staying healthy does each show?

3 Greek visitors to Rome thought that the Roman approach to public health was marvellous. Why do you think that Greeks were surprised by Roman public health? In your answer show your knowledge both of Greek and Roman medicine.

☑ **EXAM TIP**

When questions ask you to 'describe' something, include as much relevant detail you can – this will gain you more marks.

enquiry

Why was Galen so important?

One of the most influential doctors in history was called Claudius Galen. His writings shaped the way people thought about medicine for 1500 years.

Galen's use of publicity

In his early days in Rome he attracted publicity by carrying out public experiments on animals. He was an amazingly prolific writer who produced many medical books. Galen's position as doctor to the emperors greatly helped him win further publicity for his ideas.

Biography

Galen: A life

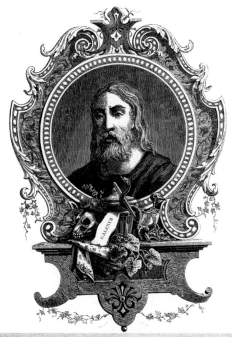

Galen was born in about AD130 in a place called Pergamon, which today is in Turkey. Pergamon was a Greek-speaking part of the Roman Empire. Galen's father was a rich architect, and Galen was well educated. His father had a dream in which the god Asklepios visited him. As a result he encouraged his son to become a doctor. Galen studied medicine in the leading medical schools of Alexandria in Egypt. In AD157 he returned home and became doctor to the gladiators of Pergamon. This was a useful experience for someone who was thinking about how the body worked. In AD161 or 162 Galen took a brave decision; he decided to move to Rome. He was well known in Pergamon but in Rome he was unheard of. His gamble paid off. He was very successful and soon many rich Romans were his patients. In AD169, the son of the emperor became his patient. In the 30 years that followed until his death in AD201 Galen was doctor to the ruling family, and the single most successful doctor in the empire.

▲ **SOURCE A** Galen is one of the most significant figures in the history of medicine. During his lifetime he was very skilful at attracting publicity for his ideas.

Galen and Greek medicine

Galen was greatly influenced by Hippocratic ideas; he also adapted the earlier Greek medical thinking. He accepted the idea of the Four Humours. Like the Hippocratic doctors he carried out careful clinical observations. However, he was ready to make changes to Hippocratic teaching. Hippocrates had suggested that often the best remedy was to let nature take its course. Galen developed more active treatments. He called for the use of 'opposites': treating symptoms with 'opposite' substances. For example, he gave pepper to patients who were too cold and cucumber to those who were too hot. Galen was also a great believer in the power of blood-letting. The Hippocratic doctors had advised that patients with fevers should be left alone and not eat. Galen rejected this advice and called for blood-letting.

Galen increased the emphasis doctors put on blood-letting. He often recommended bleeding even in cases where the patient had already lost blood through a wound or illness.

Galen and anatomy

Knowledge of anatomy had been a relatively weak area of Hippocratic medicine and Galen was determined to make it better. In Rome he was not allowed to dissect human bodies for religious reasons. Instead, Galen cut up the bodies of dead apes and pigs. He carried out public experiments on pigs in which he cut the nerves in the neck. These nerves controlled the pig's capacity to squeal. Once the nerves were cut, the pigs fell silent.

Although Galen increased anatomical knowledge his dependence on animals, rather than humans, led him to make mistakes:

- Galen's dissection of animals led him to think wrongly that the human brain was linked to a network of nerves and vessels.

- He incorrectly identified a connection between the liver and the stomach.

- Galen wrongly stated that blood moved from the right to the left ventricles of the heart via invisible pores.

Medicine after Galen

Galen was an innovator. He respected the work of Hippocrates but thought that he could improve it. He used experimentation to increase medical knowledge. Ironically, after his death Galen became established as a faultless, inspired writer who could do no wrong. It was over a thousand years before new writers challenged Galen and pointed out some of the mistakes that he had made. The early sixteenth century doctor Sylvius, was a great believer in Galen. He wrote that 'Hippocrates and Galen had never written anything that was not entirely true.' He said that if a dissection ever showed evidence contrary to Galen then there must be something wrong with the corpse!

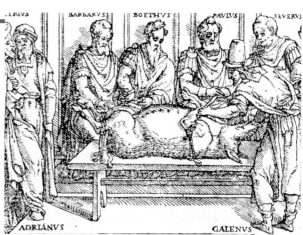

▲ **SOURCE B** Galen dissecting a pig. Unable to dissect human bodies, Galen relied on animal dissections and this led him to make some mistakes in his thinking about the human body.

QUESTIONS

1 Explain in your own words what Galen said about:

- the treatment of disease

- anatomy.

2 Do you think Galen's new treatments were an improvement on the methods used by earlier Hippocratic doctors? Explain your answer.

3 Why did Galen make so many mistakes?

4 Why is Galen important in the development of medicine?

☑ **EXAM TIP**

Make sure you write about Galen's importance, both during his own lifetime and also how he affected medicine for over 1,000 years.

Galen in his own

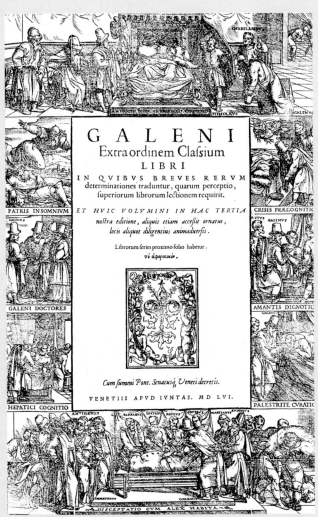

▲ **SOURCE A** This printed edition of Galen's works was published almost 1500 years after his death. Why did Galen remain so influential for so long?

> *Once I examined the skeleton of an executed robber which was lying by the side of the road. If you do not have the luck to see anything like this, you can dissect an ape and learn each of the bones by carefully removing the flesh. For this, you must choose apes which most resemble men. These are apes which do not have prominent jaws or large canine teeth. In apes like this which walk and run on two legs, you will find the same parts as in men.*

▲ **SOURCE B**

QUESTIONS

1 Look at these extracts from the writings of Galen. Where can you find evidence to support the following statements about Galen?:
   * Galen carried out careful clinical observation in line with Hippocratic ideas.
   * Galen was a scientist who believed that doctors should look carefully at the body.
   * Galen was very arrogant and thought that he was a genius.
   * Galen carried out experiments on live animals.
   * Galen found it difficult to look at the inside of the human body and had to dissect animals instead.
   * Galen treated diseases according to his theory of opposites.

2 Are these sources useful for historians carrying out the following enquiries?:
   a an enquiry into the impact of Galen on the work of other doctors
   b an enquiry into the way Galen himself worked as a doctor
   c an enquiry into Galen's reputation during his own lifetime.

3 'These sources are useful for historians of medicine but they are not necessarily reliable.' Do you agree with this statement? Explain your answer.

words

You should dissect the spinal cord of a live pig in the following way. Get a large sharp knife. The animal should be young so that it will be easy to cut through the vertebrae. Once you have opened the spinal cord, you can paralyse the body below this point by completely cutting the spinal cord. If you cut the cord near the thoraci vertebrae then the animal's breathing and squealing will be affected. Similarly, if you cut behind the fifth vertebrae both arms are paralysed.

▲ SOURCE C

I have done as much for medicine as the Emperor Trajan did for the Roman Empire when he built bridges and roads through Italy. It is I, and I alone, who have revealed the true path of medicine. It must be admitted that Hippocrates already marked out the path. He prepared the way but I have made it passable.

▲ SOURCE D

The great writer, Glaucon was full of admiration when he saw me at work. The patient was one of his friends, a Sicilian. As we entered the house of the patient, one of his friends, a servant walked past carrying a basin from the patient's room on the way to the dung heap. I pretended not to notice but I saw that it was full of human excrement looking like shreds of flesh, together with blood and pus. This is unmistakeable evidence of liver disease. Glaucon and I went into the patient's room. I took his pulse. He told me that he had recently got out of bed to go to the toilet. I put my hand on his right side and said, 'The disease is here.' The patient thought I'd worked this out just by taking his pulse and he looked at me with admiration. I said, 'You will also have a shallow, dry cough.' Almost as soon as I got the words out of my mouth he coughed in just this manner.

▲ SOURCE E

Doctors must be familiar with human bones. It is not enough to read about bones in books. You must also get to know each bone through the use of your own eyes, handling each bone for itself.

▲ SOURCE F

Something really amazing happened the first time I treated the Emperor Marcus Aurelius. Three doctors had watched him since dawn and all three said that a fever was coming. I took his pulse. Far from indicating a fever, the pulse told me that his stomach was stuffed with food, and this had become a slimy excrement. The Emperor praised my diagnosis and said over and over, 'That is it. It is just as you say. I have eaten too much cold food.' He asked what should be done. I replied, 'Usually I prescribe wine with pepper. In this case it will be enough to place a woollen cover on your stomach, soaked in hot spices.'

▲ SOURCE G

✓ EXAM TIP

Make sure you read all the questions carefully before you start to write. Question 1 helps you to practise extraction of information. Question 2 helps you to understand that different sources are useful in different ways. Question 3 shows you that sources can be useful even if you cannot trust what they say.

enquiry

What impact did the Romans have on public health in Britain?

Britain became part of the Roman world in 43 AD when the Emperor Claudius sent a Roman army to conquer the island. In places, the Celtic people of Britain resisted fiercely and the Romans were never able to secure complete control of northern Britain.

The Romans' standard approach to newly conquered lands was to get the local ruling class on their side. The Roman historian, Tacitus tells how an early governor of Britannia called Agricola used the advantages of the Roman lifestyle in order to win over influential Britons:

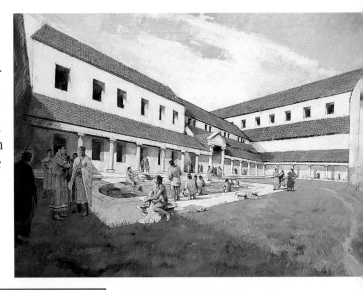

▲ SOURCE A This reconstruction picture shows the outdoor exercise yard and swimming pool at the baths in Wroxeter. Were Roman baths like this really popular with people in Roman Britain?

His purpose was to introduce them to a life of peace and quiet by the provision of facilities. And so the population was gradually led into the demoralising temptations of arcades, baths and sumptuous banquets. The unsuspecting Britons spoke of such novelties as 'civilisation', when in fact they were only a feature of their enslavement.

▲ SOURCE B Tacitus, writing in the early second century AD.

The public bath-house

Throughout the Empire the facilities of a Roman town included public bath-houses, a system for ensuring fresh water in towns and efficient sewers. There is evidence for each of these public health amenities in the towns of Roman Britain. It is important, however, to remember that Britain was a particularly remote, obscure part of the Roman Empire. It would be surprising, therefore, if public health facilities existed on the same scale as in the heart of the Empire.

The Roman Army was important in Britain. Bath-houses and military hospitals were soon built at the legionary headquarters. Military latrines can still be seen today at Housesteads, on Hadrian's Wall. This toilet block was placed on the edge of the fort up against a wall. A deep sewer washed the waste away and took it outside the fort. Unfortunately it only seems to have worked well after heavy rain and a large water tank was added to help flush the latrines. A separate water channel was used for washing the sponges that were used instead of toilet paper. After a while this channel did not work properly and static water tanks were used instead.

Archaeologists have identified the sites of public bath-houses in most towns of Roman Britain. As in the rest of the empire, people of all backgrounds, including slaves, would have been able to use the baths for a very small charge. The baths were used for a wide range of fitness activities, including athletics, ball-games and massage. At Caerleon, in Wales, archaeologists have excavated evidence that substantial amounts of shell-fish were eaten by users of the baths. People presumably ate these snacks as they chatted with their friends.

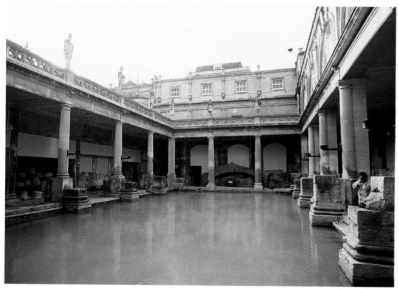

▲ **SOURCE C** The baths complex at Bath was very impressive. This was not a public health facility. It was a religious healing centre.

Perhaps the most famous bath facilities in Roman Britain were in the city of Bath. This was very different from most public bath-houses because it was essentially a religious healing centre.

Sewerage systems

British towns had less sophisticated water supply, drainage and sewerage systems than many continental Roman towns. Underground pipes for sewerage have been discovered in York, Lincoln and Colchester, however, most towns only had open sewers. York was a particularly important city, and on one occasion it was the home of the emperor himself. So it was fitting that York should have a particularly grand sanitation system. The main sewer in York was so large that slaves could enter it from manholes in order to clean and repair it. This was unusual. In another town, Silchester, there is no evidence of any kind of sewerage system and it seems that waste was simply thrown into local streams. Even the magnificent sewers of York had their problems; in the summer the flow of water was not strong enough to flush away all the waste.

Water supply

Britain does not have the same problems with water supply found in many hot dry Mediterranean countries. Perhaps this is why there are no remains in Britain that compare with the great aqueducts of Spain or southern France. Nevertheless, open conduits that brought fresh water to the towns were a standard feature of town life in Roman Britain. At Lincoln clay pipes coated with concrete brought the water 20 miles (32 kilometres). The water supply to Wroxeter was 9 million litres a day. This was a considerable achievement but we should not imagine that the towns had anything like a modern water supply. Private houses were not usually supplied with water. The skeletons of most women from a cemetery in Cirencester show common damage to the bones of the neck that was probably caused by heavy work carrying water pots.

QUESTIONS

1 According to Tacitus why did the Romans introduce public baths to Britain?

2 What other reasons are suggested for the introduction of Roman public amenities?

3 How does archaeological evidence help us to understand the nature of Roman public health in Britain?

enquiry

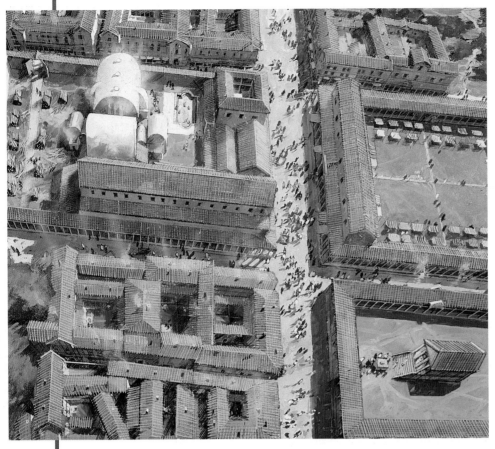

Toilets

Roman towns were provided with public toilets. Archaeologists in St Alban's have located the site of some public toilets. These had room for ten people. There were no cubicles and no privacy. Remarkably, in York, some of the toilet sponges have survived and have been excavated by archaeologists working on the town's sewerage system. People did not usually have toilets or privies in their houses. Instead, they used pots that were then taken outside and emptied into sewers or streams.

◄ **SOURCE A** The public baths were at the centre of the town of Wroxeter. Strangely, the baths were abandoned before the end of the Roman period.

The demise of public health facilities

Archaeologists have discovered a puzzling fact relating to the final century of Roman rule in Britain. In many ways the fourth century AD seems to have been a time of great peace and prosperity for Roman Britain. At the same time, the public health facilities in the towns were beginning to fall apart. The public baths were demolished in Canterbury in the fourth century. Grass and weeds were growing in the baths in Exeter. The baths at Wroxeter were abandoned many years before the end of Roman rule.

How good was Roman public health in Britain? Different archaeological interpretations

Modern historians disagree about the impact of Roman public health. Look at the following extracts from some of their writings.

The impression given by most descriptions of town life in the Roman Empire is of spacious, well-organised streets, water on tap, an efficient sewerage system; but this may not be the whole picture or even an accurate one. The great civic bath-houses, unless kept scrupulously clean, would have been hotbeds of disease. Housewives had to carry water from public water tanks or draw it from a well. Sewers were often open or built very close to the surface, leading to unpleasant smells and disease.

▲ **SOURCE B** Lindsay Allason-Jones, *Women in Roman Britain*, 1989.

SOURCE C ▶
A reconstruction picture of the legionary latrine at Housesteads.

In Britain, in towns like Chichester, Leicester and Wroxeter in Shropshire, probably as many as 500 people a day used the baths.

Water in most large towns in Britain was supplied by aqueducts. The most impressive surviving example is in Dorchester; an eight-mile channel, 5 feet wide (1.6 metres) and more than 3 feet (1 metre) deep. The aqueduct at Wroxeter could deliver 2 million gallons of water each day.

◀ SOURCE D Keith Branigan, *Roman Britain*, 1980.

Bathing would have been entirely new to most of the British population and it does not seem to have been a major priority. The bath-house at Exeter was demolished after AD 85. What would appear to be a desirable facility was torn down. This implies a lack of enthusiasm about public baths. Curiously at Wroxeter public baths begun in the late first century were knocked down, while still incomplete.

There is very little evidence for water being made available for use by individuals in Britain. Even in the major towns water pipes or aqueducts are normally only associated with baths. Most people would have been accustomed to taking water from wells and rivers.

▲ SOURCE E Guy de la Bedoyère *Roman Towns in Britain*, 1992.

QUESTIONS

1 Explain how archaeologists disagree about public health in Roman Britain.

2 What impact did the Romans have on public health in Britain? Include the following points when answering the question:

- the facilities they built

- how they were actually used.

Finish by making your own judgement.

review

Prehistory to the ancient world

How much change was there in medicine? Supernatural to natural approaches

Look back at your work on prehistoric and Aborigine medicine and think about the aspects that relied on supernatural/religious ideas, and the aspects that were practical/non-supernatural. Summarise your ideas in table form like the one shown on the right. Some of the table has already been completed for you:

Prehistoric and Aborigine Medicine	
Supernatural/ religious	Practical/ non-supernatural
Trephination took place; it may have been to get rid of demons.	Aborigines had a good knowledge of many herbal remedies.

In discussing the ancient world you need to show knowledge and understanding of Egyptian, Greek and Roman medicine. Progress was made in each society, but in different areas of medical knowledge. In all three societies people developed natural, non-superstitious approaches to medical problems. Alongside these natural approaches, supernatural explanations continued to exist.

Write the following statements in the correct place under three headings in a table (like the one shown below) from left to right across a double page. You will need to look back at what you have learned about the different ancient civilizations to identify what statement goes where and the person that is sometimes being referred to.

Aspects of medicine	Egyptian medicine	Greek medicine	Roman medicine
Anatomy & Surgery			
Public Health			
Doctors & Healing			
Diseases & Treatments			

A There is evidence that their doctors began to specialise in treating particular diseases or parts of the body.

B Their doctors had a clear sense of their duty to the patient which was summed up in the Oath they took.

C Later Greek doctors moved here and established the idea of the professional doctor. These Greek doctors were often disliked.

D Anatomical knowledge increased during this period.

E Their wealth allowed people for the first time to work as full-time doctors.

F He increased anatomical knowledge but his research on animals rather than humans led him to make several important mistakes.

G At this time there was a divide between the supernatural approach found in the temple and the natural approach of the doctors.

H Their engineering skills provided spectacular aqueducts in some parts of their Empire.

I He was a Greek doctor working in the Roman Empire.

J   In the early days there were no professional doctors; the head of each family took responsibility for medicine.

K   His writings influenced doctors for over a thousand years.

L   They worked out a basic knowledge of the internal organs of the body and that they were connected by blood vessels.

M   Early on their doctors had little interest in anatomy or surgery because they believed 'nature was the best healer'.

N   These people used both natural and supernatural explanations of disease, and their treatments combined the two approaches.

O   These people continued the Greek situation; patients could find both natural and supernatural treatments.

P   The doctors at Alexandria in the third century BC specialised in anatomy.

Q   Public Health was not a priority for either of these two peoples. In both these societies the government did not take steps to help the poor to prevent illness.

R   Rich people looked after their own welfare and health in both these societies.

S   The approach of the government was to look after its citizens by the provision of fresh, clean water and sanitation.

T   They did carry out blood-letting.

U   They learned a lot from their sacrifice of animals and less from their religious beliefs about the afterlife.

☑ EXAM TIP

Make sure you understand that natural ideas about medicine did not completely replace the older supernatural ideas and that both continued side-by-side.

The Ancient World and the factors for change

Individuals: Can you add any more information about the part the following individuals played in the development of medicine?
- *Aristotle: a biologist who made careful observation of animals; he identified the key part played by the heart.*
- *Hippocrates: his followers rejected supernatural explanations for disease; the Hippocratic doctors believed in the Four Humours; they carefully observed their patients.*
- *Galen: increased medical knowledge by carrying out experiments on animals; he developed the theory of treating symptoms with an 'opposite' remedy; he made a number of mistakes because he found it difficult to study the inside of the human body.*

Government: Look back at your work on Egypt and Rome. What impact did strong governments have on medicine in these different societies?

Religion: Look back at your work on Egypt and Greece. What impact did powerful religious beliefs have on medicine in these different societies?

War: Look back at your work on Rome. What influence did the Roman army have upon medical provision in the empire?

Science: Look back at your work on Egypt and Greece. What impact did careful observation have on medicine in their different societies?

overview

Welcome to the Middle Ages

Timeline

476 — Last Roman emperor in the west of Europe is overthrown

632–700 — Islamic armies establish a new Islamic empire

1258 — Baghdad is destroyed by an invading Mongol army and the last Caliph is killed

1348 — The Black Death arrives in Europe

1445 — The first printed book is produced in Europe

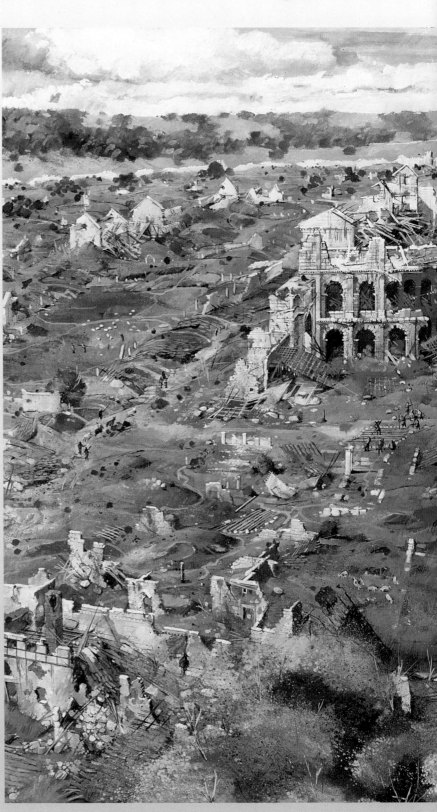

The Roman Empire in most of Europe collapsed in the fifth century. The Empire had been under attack for some time from tribes of barbarians who had gathered on its northern and eastern frontiers. The barbarians eventually overran the Empire in a series of invasions.

After the collapse of the Roman Empire there was no longer a single government throughout most of Europe. Instead power lay in the hands of the kings and chieftains who controlled the barbarian tribes. They were warriors who loved fighting and warfare. As a result there were **frequent wars** between the different barbarian groups.

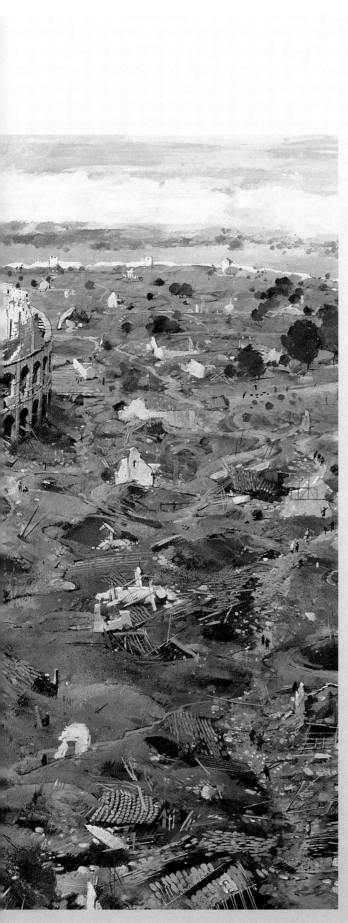

The new rulers did not share the Roman ideas about the **role of government**. The Romans thought that the government had a responsibility for the health and welfare of citizens. The barbarian kings and chieftains had no such ideas about government. For them the job of a ruler was to fight, not to look after people's welfare.

The fall of Rome also led to a **collapse in the economy**. Roman money no longer circulated. Under the Romans the currency had been used by most people and was essential for the wealth and success of the economy. The Roman road system also broke down. As a result of these changes people became much poorer. Flourishing industries, such as pottery making, disintegrated.

When they first arrived, the barbarian tribes were non-Christians. They worshipped their own gods. They were soon converted to Christianity. Barbarian chieftains and kings relied upon priests because they could read and write and were well educated. **The Church**, therefore, became more powerful even when the rest of Roman civilisation was falling apart.

☑ **EXAM TIP**

Make sure you can work out how each of these **key features** might affect medicine.

◀ **SOURCE A** The centre of the Roman city of Canterbury in the fifth century. After the departure of the Roman legionaries, towns like this were largely abandoned.

enquiry

What happened to medicine after the fall of the Roman Empire?

What were the Dark Ages?

The start of the medieval period is sometimes known as the Dark Ages. Is this a fair description in terms of medical history? There was a time of chaos in much of Europe as the Roman Empire disintegrated and was replaced by new barbarian kingdoms. There were several consequences for medicine:

- centres for the training of doctors disappeared

- many of the key books of Greek and Roman medical knowledge were destroyed and lost

- Roman public health systems collapsed.

There was no proper system for the training of doctors in the centuries after the fall of the Roman Empire. Some people claimed to be 'doctors' but they had not experienced a thorough medical education. The doctors of the Dark Ages made little use of the writings of the Greeks and the Romans. Instead, they relied on a mixture of practical remedies and superstition. Typical of these practitioners was a Frankish woman called Morigund (from modern France). We know that her remedies included treating ulcers with prayers and spit mixed with leaves or fruit. From England there are Anglo-Saxon medical books that give some commonsense folk remedies and many magical charms. This type of folk medicine had some value; one historian has identified 185 plants that were listed as having medical properties in a tenth century Anglo-Saxon text. Modern scientific analysis shows that two thirds of these plants (120 in total) would have some beneficial impact on patients.

Many of the great libraries of the Roman world were destroyed at the time of the fall of the Roman Empire. The new barbarian rulers were largely illiterate and cared little for scholarship and books. As a result many Greek and Roman medical books were lost in western Europe. These included most of the works of Galen and the Hippocratic writers. A few classical medical books were preserved in the monasteries of western Europe. These were the only centres of higher education. Books that survived included some of the key Roman herbal books, which listed plants and their medical properties. It seems that the people of the Dark Ages liked these books because they had an obvious practical value, while they were less interested in more theoretical books. The Greek and Roman idea of the Four Humours was kept alive by an influential Spanish writer called Isidore, who wrote in the early seventh century.

Throughout much of the empire the elaborate Roman systems of sanitation broke down in the fifth and sixth centuries. Public bath-houses fell into disuse. Aqueducts and sewerage systems were no longer maintained. The new barbarian rulers had neither the Roman technological knowledge nor the Roman interest in the welfare of their subjects. An eighth century Anglo-Saxon writer described, in amazement, the ruins of a Roman bath-house, almost certainly in the city of Bath:

QUESTIONS

1 Does the poet seem to know what the ruins had been used for? Explain your answer.

2 Is it fair to describe the early centuries of the medieval period as a Dark Age for medicine? In your answer you could mention:

- Folk medicine

- The preservation of Greek and Roman ideas

- The collapse of the Roman public health system

- The training of doctors.

Wondrous is this masonry, shattered by the Fates. The buildings raised by giants are crumbling. The roofs have collapsed, the towers are in ruins. Here were splendid palaces and many halls with water flowing through them. And now these rooms lie desolate. Here stood courts of stone, and a stream gushed forth in rippling floods of hot water.

▲ SOURCE A From an anonymous Anglo-Saxon poem known as 'The Ruin'.

The woman who cannot bring her child to term must go to a dead man's grave, step three times over the grave and say these words three times:
'This as my help against the evil late birth,
This as my help against the grievous dismal birth,
This is my help against the evil lame birth.'

And when that woman is with child and she goes to bed with her lord, then she must say:
'Up I go, step over you
With a live child, not with a dying one,
With a full-born child, not with a doomed one.'
And when the mother feels that the child is alive, she must go to church, and when she comes in front of the alter, then she must say:
Christ, I said, make this known!

▲ SOURCE B An Anglo-Saxon charm for pregnant women whose babies are overdue.

Medicine in the

Source Exercises

The evidence of the Venerable Bede

In the early Middle Ages there was much less writing than in the Roman period and we have fewer documents for sources. One major exception is the extensive writing of an English monk called Bede, who lived in the north-east of England in the early eighth century.

Bishop John came one day to a convent of nuns at Watton, near Beverley. The abbess said that one of her nuns, her own daughter, was very seriously ill. The sick girl was called Coenburg. The abbess said that the nun had recently been bled in the arm and, during the blood-letting, Coenburg was suddenly seized by a violent pain. Afterwards the arm became so swollen that it could hardly be encircled with two hands. Now she was in terrible pain and likely to die. When the bishop learned that the blood-letting had taken place on the fourth day of the moon he said, 'You have acted most foolishly. Don't you know that it is dangerous to bleed people when the light of the moon and the pull of the tide is increasing?' He went to see the girl and said a prayer over her, and left. The girl made a complete recovery. Later she said, 'As soon as the bishop blessed me I began to feel better. The pain entirely left my arm. It was as though the bishop took it away with him.'

▲ **SOURCE A** The Anglo-Saxon writer, Bede. What can we learn from his writings about medicine during the Dark Ages?

☑ EXAM TIP

You need to consider whether the evidence is reliable for beliefs about medicine, as well as for the events described. Use your own knowledge to help you.

Dark Ages

The physician, Cynfrid was present at the death of Ethelreda. He said that during her last illness she had a large tumour under her jaw. 'I was asked,' he said, 'to open the tumour and drain away the poison inside it. I did this, and for two days she seemed a little better. But on the third day the earlier pain returned, and she died. It is said that when she was affected by this tumour and pain in her jaw and neck, she welcomed the pain and used to say, 'I know that I deserve this painful disease on my neck because when I was a girl I used to wear jewellery around my neck. I believe that God in His goodness wishes me to endure this pain in my neck as a punishment for my needless vanity as a girl. So now I wear a burning red tumour on my neck instead of gold and pearls.'

I must tell you about a cure that took place just three years ago and was told to me by the very monk to whom it happened. A young monk developed a tumour on his eyelid, which grew every day and threatened to destroy the eye. Although the physicians applied poultices to reduce it, they had no success. Some doctors advised cutting it out, others opposed this, fearing that an operation would bring grave complications. So the brother suffered great pain for a long time, and it seemed that no human skills could prevent the loss of his eye until one day he was cured by God and the relics of Saint Cuthbert. Some hairs of the saint were kept at the monastery as a relic. The abbot gave the hairs to the young man with the diseased eye. He placed the hairs of holy Cuthbert on his eyelid, and held them there for a while. He then replaced the relics in their special casket, confident that, now that his eye had been touched by the hairs of the holy man of God, it would soon be cured. Nor was his faith in vain. Later in the day he suddenly felt his eye and found it sound, as though there had never been any deformity or swelling on it.

▲ The three extracts are from Bede's *History of the English Church and People*.

QUESTIONS

1 What do these extracts tell us about medicine? In your answer you could mention whether there is any evidence that:

   a there were doctors in the Dark Age period

   b some people believed in supernatural approaches to disease

   c some people believed in natural approaches to the treatment of disease.

2 Bede was a monk and a member of the Church. Does that make his evidence more or less reliable in any way?

Concluding your enquiry:

What happened to medicine after the fall of the Roman Empire: The Dark Ages?

- Identify examples of progress (change for the better)

- Identify examples of regress (change for the worse)

- Identify examples of little or no change

- Draw your conclusion based on your own examples.

enquiry

How did Islamic medicine contribute to medical progress?

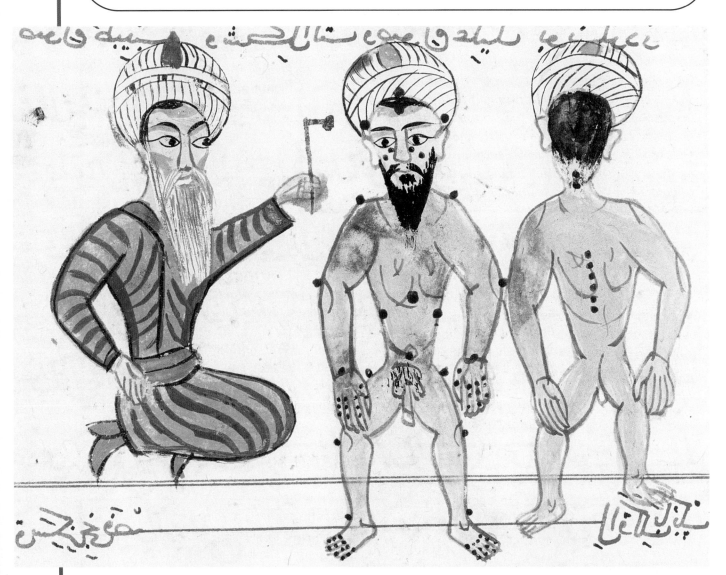

▲ **SOURCE A** An Arabic text of the Middle Ages showing the places where the doctor should apply cautery points to the patient's leprosy sores.

☑ **EXAM TIP**

Make sure you can compare what happened in medicine in western Europe with what happened in the Islamic Empire.

While the collapse of the Roman Empire led to chaos in western Europe, the history of medicine in the Middle East was entirely different. In the seventh century AD the followers of the Prophet Muhammad established an enormous new Islamic Empire in the Middle East and North Africa. During the following centuries Islamic doctors made a great contribution to medical knowledge.

The success of the Islamic doctors depended on government support. For several centuries the Islamic Empire was a single state ruled over by one man, known as the Caliph. The Caliph provided the stability needed for medical progress. Many Caliphs were interested in science. During the reign of Caliph Harun al-Rashid (AD 786–809), a centre for the translation of Greek manuscripts into Arabic was set up in Baghdad (the capital of the Islamic empire and now the capital of modern Iraq). This initiative preserved hundreds of precious manuscripts. The translated manuscripts included the major works of Hippocrates and Galen, forgotten in western Europe.

Caliph Harun also set up a major new hospital in Baghdad in about AD805. In contrast with Christian hospitals of the Middle Ages, this was intended to offer treatment, and not simply care, to patients. A medical school and library were set up as part of the hospital. Soon other similar hospitals, called 'bimaristans', were built in many other cities of the Islamic empire. These hospitals provided medical care for all: men and women, rich and poor, Muslim and non-Muslim. Doctors were permanently present and medical students were given training by working alongside these physicians.

It was in the Islamic world that the first hospitals specifically for people with mental illnesses were set up. These were called 'maristans'. In contrast with medieval Christians, Islamic doctors did not see people with mental illness as being possessed by spirits. Instead the mentally ill were treated with compassion as victims of an unfortunate illness.

▼ SOURCE B A map of the Middle East in the eleventh century, showing Islamic States.

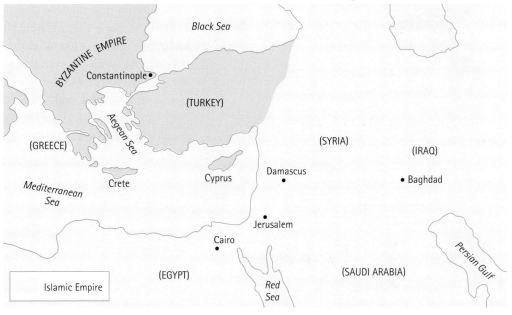

enquiry

The outbreak of smallpox begins with a continued fever, pain in the back, itching in the nose and terrors in the sleep.

These are the specific symptoms of its start:

- *a pain in the back with fever;*
- *a pricking which the patient feels all over his body;*
- *an inflamed colour, and vivid redness in both cheeks;*
- *redness of both the eyes:*
- *heaviness of the whole body;*
- *a pain in the throat and chest, with slight difficulty in breathing and cough;*
- *dryness of the breath, thick spittle and hoarseness of the voice;*
- *pain and heaviness of the head;*
- *nausea and anxiety.*

Nausea and anxiety are more frequent in the measles than in the smallpox; while on the other hand, the pain in the back is more typical of smallpox than the measles.

▲ **SOURCE A** The first description of smallpox from a book by Rhazes, ninth century.

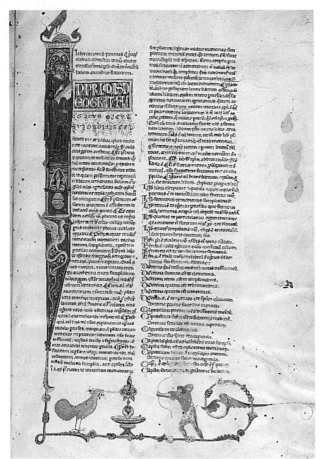

If the ninth century was a time of translation and the preservation of Greek and Roman ideas, the tenth century was a time of new medical ideas. A Persian scientist called Al-Razi (c.864–c.935) made a major contribution to medical knowledge. This influential writer was known in western Europe as Rhazes. He stressed the need for careful observation of the patient. His own careful recording enabled him to distinguish for the first time between measles and smallpox. He believed in the importance of a healthy environment. He was asked to become the first director of a new hospital in Baghdad. To find the best site for this new hospital he hung up meat in different parts of the city and compared the way the meat decayed in different places. He recommended that the hospital should be built at the place where the meat decayed the least.

The second great Islamic medical expert was Ibn Sina (980–1037), known in the West as Avicenna. Like Al-Razi, Ibn Sina was from a Persian family. He produced a great encyclopaedia of medicine known as 'al-Qanun', or 'The Canon'. This extraordinary book was a million-word summary of the whole of medical knowledge as it then was. He summarised Galen and the Hippocratic writers, together with the findings of Islamic writers. The book was amazingly comprehensive; it contained, for example, sections on anorexia and obesity. Ibn Sina, like many Islamic doctors, was particularly knowledgeable about the medical use of drugs. New drugs from the Islamic world included many substances that are still used in medicine such as camphor, laudanum, naptha and senna. The word 'drug' itself is Arabic. Ibn Sina's encyclopaedia listed the medical properties of 760 different drugs.

◄ **SOURCE B** The works of Ibn Sina were copied throughout Christian Europe. This late medieval manuscript was used by teachers at the University of Oxford, England.

The Islamic writers accepted the basic principles of Galen's work and that of the Hippocratic writers. At the same time the Islamic doctors were quite prepared to criticise the Greek and Roman authorities. Al-Razi saw himself as a disciple of Galen but he thought that all disciples should seek to improve the work of their masters. One of his books was actually called 'Doubts about Galen'. A later Islamic doctor, Ibn al-Nafis, correctly identified that Galen was wrong about how the heart worked. Galen had mistakenly stated that blood moved from the right to the left ventricles of the heart via invisible pores. Ibn al-Nafis said that this was impossible, 'The septum between the ventricles does not contain an invisible passage as Galen thought, therefore, the blood must only pass through the lungs.' He suggested for the first time the circulation of the blood round the body via the lungs. Unfortunately his book was not one of the Islamic books that was read in the West and people in Europe continued to accept Galen's mistake until the seventeenth century.

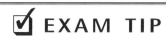

☑ EXAM TIP

Make sure you can compare what happened in medicine in western Europe with what happened in the Islamic Empire.

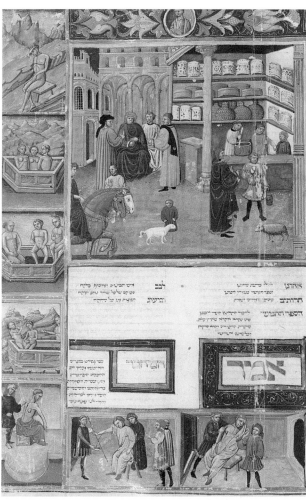

▲ SOURCE C Scene from an open-air pharmacy taken from a late medieval Middle-Eastern medical book.

QUESTIONS

1   Explain in your own words how Islamic hospitals were organised.

2   Why are Rhazes and Ibn Sina important individuals in the history of medicine?

3   'There was no medical progress for a thousand years after the collapse of the Roman Empire.' Using information from this unit explain whether you agree with this statement. In your answer you could mention:

- How Islamic scholars preserved Greek and Roman medical texts.

- How Islamic doctors developed classical ideas about medical practice and 'clinical observation'.

- How new hospitals were built, including mental hospitals.

- Research into new medical drugs.

- Criticisms of some of the errors of Galen and the Hippocratic doctors.

enquiry

What was the role of the Church in medieval medicine?

After the collapse of the Roman Empire, the Church was the only organisation in western Europe that tried to keep alive the medical ideas of Ancient Greece and Rome. Priests, monks and nuns were almost the only people who could read and write. In monasteries many precious medical manuscripts were saved from destruction.

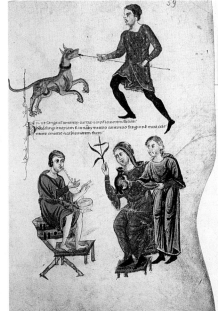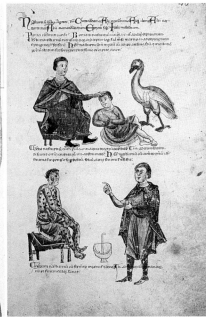

▶ **SOURCE A** Monks kept alive much Greek and Roman medical knowledge. This medical text describes how herbs can be used in treating different complaints. It was drawn by a monk in Canterbury in the eleventh century.

The Middle Ages were a very religious time and supernatural explanations of disease also remained extremely common. God and the saints in heaven were thought to intervene in daily life, either to make people sick or better. Some medical conditions, such as blindness and leprosy, were particularly seen as having been sent by God. Despite the fact that Hippocratic doctors had rejected supernatural explanations nearly 2,000 years before, epilepsy was often seen in the Middle Ages as a condition caused by God.

The Church did not encourage very positive attitudes towards those with mental illness. Those with mental problems were viewed either as possessed by devils or deliberately wicked people who needed to be punished. Throughout the Middle Ages, the Church encouraged the flogging of the mentally ill as a way of 'driving out' the demons.

Although the Church explained some illness in supernatural terms, this did not stop some members of the Church from taking practical steps to help sick people get better. Before the thirteenth century, many priests and other clergy were also doctors. The English royal family, for example, relied upon priests and monks for their medical care before 1200. William the Conqueror's doctor was Baldwin, abbot of Bury St Edmund's Abbey. One priest-doctor, called Peter of Spain, became Pope (overall leader of the Church) in 1276.

Christianity brought a new idea to medical care in western Europe. This was the belief that it was particularly good to help other people who were neglected by society, including the poorest sick people, who could not look after themselves. Care for such people was seen as a way of imitating Christ. St Jerome, one of the most influential early Christian writers described with great approval a rich woman called Fabiola, 'She gathered together all the sick from the streets and personally tended the victims of hunger and disease. I have often seen her washing wounds which others could hardly bare to look at.' This commitment to the service of others was quite different to earlier Greek and Roman medical tradition.

The care for the poor and sick led the Church to set up many hospitals during the Middle Ages. Almost all medieval hospitals in Europe were run by the Church. The Hotel Dieu in Paris was founded in the seventh century. It still exists today and is the oldest working hospital in the world. There was a great expansion of hospitals in the eleventh to fourteenth centuries. Throughout England and Wales 1,100 hospitals were set up during the Middle Ages. These hospitals varied greatly in size. Many were extremely small. It was common for them to be limited to no more than twelve patients, in memory of the twelve disciples of Jesus. A few were very large. St. Leonard's, in York, was unusually large and could look after 200 sick people.

A great leprosy epidemic in the twelfth and thirteenth centuries stimulated the growth of hospital care by the Church. Specialist leper hospitals were built throughout Europe. One calculation is that there were 19,000 leper hospitals by 1225. Some of these leper houses were also used to isolate plague victims during the Black Death. Later specialist 'pest houses' were built for those with the plague or suspected of being infected.

Medieval Christian hospitals were very different from modern hospitals. They looked after the poor as well as the sick. The emphasis was on care and religion rather than treatment and cure. As a result doctors were not particularly important people in many medieval hospitals. The staff of the large hospital of St Leonard's in York had several chaplains but no doctor. St Bartholomew's Hospital in London was founded in 1123. It was nearly 500 years later that a permanent doctor was appointed to the hospital in the sixteenth century. The original staff were brothers and sisters in religious orders who cared for the sick and tried to save their souls, but did not attempt to cure them. Hospitals in France and Italy were more advanced than those in Britain. A doctor was appointed to the Hotel Dieu in Paris, in 1231, many centuries before the doctor at St Bartholomew's.

The medieval Church was a very conservative organisation. The leaders of the Church were not usually interested in new ideas and were suspicious of change. The dissection of the human body was not formally forbidden by the Church, but the Church discouraged this kind of experimentation. People who did try to develop new scientific ideas sometimes got into trouble with the Church. Roger Bacon, a leading scientist, was imprisoned for many years because the Church was unhappy with his experiments.

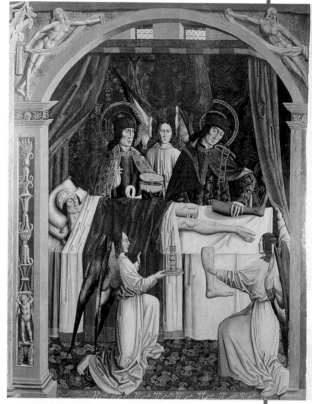

▲ **SOURCE B** The Church taught that saints could heal sick people through miracles. This painting shows saints Cosmas and Damian helped by angels miraculously replacing a sick white man's leg with the leg from a dead black man.

QUESTION

'The medieval Church only encouraged people to take supernatural approaches to medical problems.' Do you agree with this statement? In your answer:

- say whether there is evidence that the Church used supernatural approaches

- say whether there is evidence of non-supernatural approaches

- give a balanced conclusion.

The medieval Ch

What was the medieval Church's attitude to the sick?

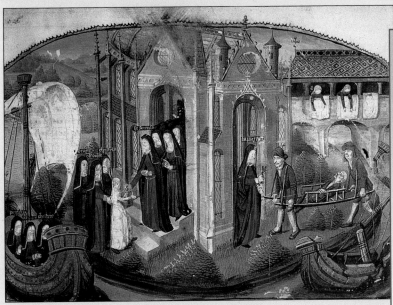

▲ SOURCE A A patient arriving at a medieval hospital and being greeted by a nun. In the background nuns clean the hospital's bed clothes.

Healing shrines flourished, and scores of saints were invoked each organ of the body and each complaint had a particular saint: St Artemis for genital afflictions; St Roch protected against plague buboes; St Lawrence for backache,' St Bernardine for the lungs, St Vitus for chorea (St Vitus's dance) and St Fiacre for sore arses. St Apollonia became the patron saint of toothache because all her teeth had been knocked out during her martyrdom.

▲ SOURCE B Professor Roy Porter worked for the Wellcome Institute for the History of Medicine in London. This extract is from his book, *The Greatest Benefit to Mankind* (1997).

Although primarily concerned with the spiritual health of their patients, medieval hospitals aimed to provide a clean, calm atmosphere, in which rest, regular meals and careful nursing would either hasten recovery or lessen the suffering of the terminally ill.

▲ SOURCE C Carole Rawcliffe, *Medicine and Society in Later Medieval England* (1995).

When the body of St Martin was carried in procession it healed all the sick who met the procession. Now there were near the church two wandering beggars, one was blind and the other could not walk. One said to the other, 'See, the body of St Martin is now being borne in procession, and if it catches up with us we shall be healed immediately, and no one in the future will give us any money, but we shall have to work.' Then the blind man said to the lame man, 'Get up on my shoulders because I am strong, and you who see well can guide me.' They did this and tried to escape but the procession overtook them, and because of the crowd they were not able to get away. So they were healed against their will.

▲ SOURCE D Jacques de Vitry, a French priest and writer, described this incident in a sermon he preached in the thirteenth century.

rch and medicine

The infirmary of your convent must be equipped with everything necessary for looking after the sick. Medicine must be provided, and this is best done if the sister in charge has some knowledge of medicine. One of the sisters should know about blood letting, otherwise it will be necessary for a man to come in to the convent for this purpose.

▲ **SOURCE E** Peter Abelard, a French priest and teacher, writing in the early twelfth century.

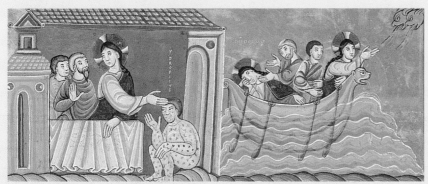

▲ **SOURCE G** St Roch was the patron saint of plague victims. In this picture an angel points to the saint's own plague sores.

The work in this hospital is extremely hard, as day and night the sick must be tended, cleaned up, put to bed, bathed, dried, fed, given drinks, carried from one bed to another and lifted. Some patients are hard to look after and impossible to please. They abuse the sisters with foul language, while others, who are mad from their sickness, strike and wound the sisters.

▲ **SOURCE H** A late medieval account of the work of the nuns at the Hotel Dieu Hospital in Paris.

▼ **SOURCE F** *The Rule of St Benedict*, sixth century. The Rule of St Benedict was the single most important guide to the way monasteries should be organised.

*Above all things,
care must be taken of the sick,
and they should be looked after as if they were Christ in person;
There should be a special room for the sick
The sick should be given baths as often as they need.*

☑ **EXAM TIP**

Selecting different evidence can lead to conflicting interpretations.

QUESTIONS

1 Sources B and C are modern interpretations. Do they take a positive or a negative view of the Church and medieval medicine?

2 Do the other sources support a positive or negative view?

3 'The Christian Church was concerned with the care rather than the cure of the sick.' Use all the sources and your background knowledge in your answer. You may wish to refer to:

- mental illness
- hospitals
- caring for the sick
- doctors and their work
- the causes of illness
- medical discoveries and progress

Concluding your enquiry:
What was the role of the Church in Medieval medicine?
- Consider how the Church helped the care of the sick
- Consider how the Church hindered progress
- Consider how the Church used supernatural methods
- Choose the most important feature to conclude your enquiry.

enquiry

Was progress made in medicine during the Middle Ages?

Medieval explanations of disease

The following source was written in England in the fifteenth century but it reflects an explanation of disease that was established almost 2,000 years earlier in Ancient Greece. What evidence can you find in the source of the continuing impact of Ancient Greek ideas?

> *Now in every man's body are four qualities: hot or cold, moist or dry. The amount of heat or cold is the cause of the colour of urine. Too much heat in the body makes the urine red. Moistness or dryness determine how thick or thin the urine is. If the patient's urine is, for example, red and thick it means that the blood is too hot and moist. If urine is red and thin this shows that choler is too hot and dry. If the urine appears white this is a sign of too much phlegm because phlegm is cold and moist. If the urine is white and thin it is a sign of too much melancholy for melancholy is cold and dry.*

▲ **SOURCE B** Text from a fifteenth century Urine chart.

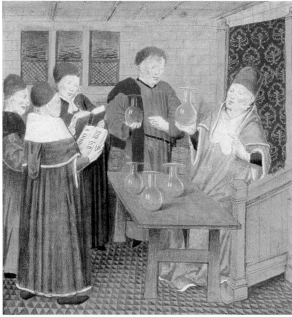

▲ **SOURCE A** A doctor and his assistants inspect the urine of a patient. The patient is not present. Belief in the usefulness of urine inspection was so strong that some doctors did not bother to meet the patients.

You have probably spotted that Source B shows a continuing belief in the Hippocratic idea of the Four Humours. Explanations of disease changed very little during the Middle Ages. Medieval doctors accepted the Greek idea of the Four Humours and believed that an imbalance of humours was often the cause of illness. The main means of diagnosis was 'uroscopy', the study of urine through the use of the doctor's senses of sight, smell and taste. The greatest praise that you could give to a medieval doctor, was to describe him or her as a great judge of urine. Some doctors were so convinced of the power of urine inspection that they did not bother to meet the patient. Instead they sent an assistant to visit the patient and collect the all-important urine sample.

Medieval people had other explanations of disease. We have seen in the unit on the role of the Church (pages 64–65) that many people looked to religious or supernatural explanations for disease. Towards the end of the Middle Ages there was a great increase in the popularity of astrological ideas. According to astrology, the health of people was influenced by the position of the stars and the planets. This was not an alternative to the Four Humours; late medieval doctors believed both in the balance of the humours and the influence of the heavens.

Healers

The training of the doctors who served the wealthy was increasingly well organised in the Middle Ages. In the twelfth century, universities were set up for the first time and they began to train doctors and to give them examinations before they qualified. Some universities were particularly famous for their medical schools, including Montpellier in France and Bologna in northern Italy.

One negative result of the rise of the universities was that women doctors found it increasingly difficult to practice. The universities were strictly for men only. Most European universities did not open their doors to women until the late nineteenth and early twentieth centuries. The system of educating and licensing doctors through university qualifications led to women being left out of this part of medicine. In 1322, for example, there is a case from Paris of the university accusing a women called Jacoba of working as a doctor without proper qualifications. She was put on trial by the university. Many contented patients gave evidence saying how skilful she was. Despite this, Jacoba was found guilty of practising medicine although unqualified and fined the then huge sum of £60.

While women were banned from university medicine schools, they continued to be heavily involved in the provision of medical care for the majority of poor people who could not afford a university-trained doctor. Women also continued to work as midwives. The university doctors disliked women doctors. The rise of the university schools of medicine led to many arguments between doctors and other medical workers. In particular, the university doctors saw themselves as superior to **apothecaries** and to **barber-surgeons**.

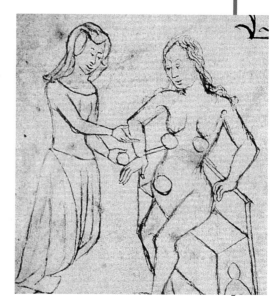

▲ **SOURCE C** A woman healer draws blood by 'cupping' a woman patient.

QUESTIONS

1   How does Source B show that Hippocratic ideas were still believed in the late Middle Ages?

2   How did medieval doctors use the inspection of urine to work out the causes of sickness? Can you use this information to explain what is going on in Source A?

3   In what way was increasing use made of astrology in the late Middle Ages?

4   How did the coming of universities change the way doctors were trained?

5   What was the impact of the new university schools of medicine on women who wanted to be doctors?

6   Look at the following list of developments in medieval medicine. For each one explain whether or not it indicated progress in medicine:

   a   belief in the Four Humours

   b   use of urine inspection

   c   increase in astrology

   d   new university schools of medicine.

KEY WORDS

apothecary –	a person who sells medical drugs
barber-surgeon –	a person who combined shaving and hairdressing with simple surgical operations

enquiry

Doctors at work

Medieval doctors were great believers in preventive medicine. They often gave helpful, practical advice about ways of keeping the Four Humours in balance.

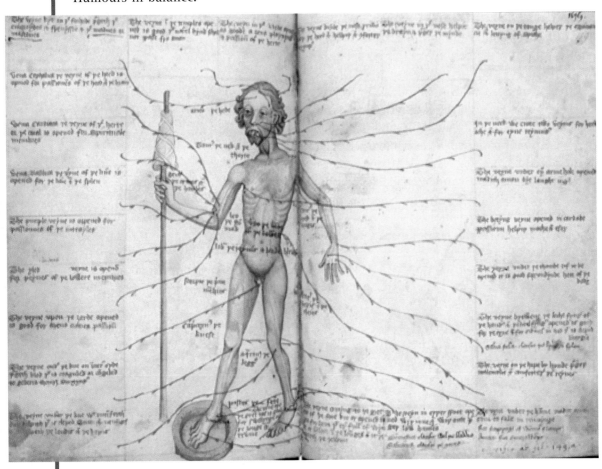

◀ SOURCE D
A blood letting man. This fifteenth-century chart shows all the places where doctors could cut the patient in order to draw blood. What was the purpose of the staff the patient is holding?

Keep your head warm. Eat no raw meat. Drink wholesome wine. Don't overeat. Don't drink alcohol just before you go to bed. A sensible diet will give you kindly digestion and golden sleep. This will keep the four humours in balance.

▲ SOURCE E John Lydgate *Dietary and Doctrine for the Pestilence*, Fifteenth century.

One aspect of preventive medicine that was of less practical value was the custom of blood-letting. People had their blood removed when they were perfectly healthy as a way of keeping the humours in balance. We can tell from the detailed records kept by monasteries that monks usually underwent blood-letting six or seven times a year. Blood-letting was seen as a treat by many monks and nuns because they were given three days off their church duties while they recovered.

Blood-letting was carried out by barber-surgeons. Some of these were not very skilful. People sometimes bled to death as a result of incompetent blood-letting. For example, an inquest held in London, in 1278, recorded how William le Paumer, a skinner by trade, had collapsed and died after his body was weakened by blood-letting. It seems that an artery had been accidentally cut!

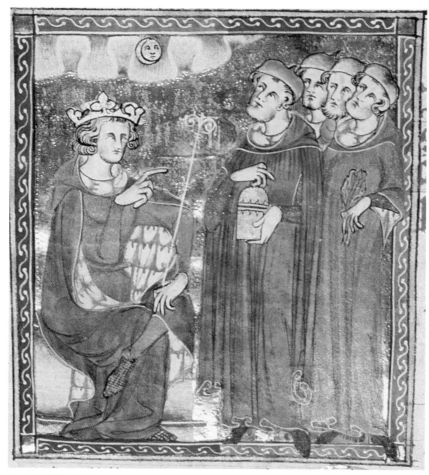

▲ **SOURCE F** Emptying the bowels was an important treatment. This fourteenth-century picture shows doctors presenting laxatives to a king. They are looking to the moon to work out the best time to take the laxatives.

The standard means of blood-letting was 'venesection' – cutting a vein. Women, children and the elderly often had blood taken through 'cupping'. The skin was scratched so that blood was drawn. Then a hot cup was placed on the graze, as it cooled this led to the gentle drawing of blood.

Blood-letting was used not only to prevent disease but also to restore health to those who were ill. Medieval doctors recommended other treatments to bring the humours back into balance. Sometimes hot baths were ordered as a way of steaming out impurities. Patients were frequently given laxatives to restore balance by emptying the bowels. Some doctors made great use of enemas for the same purpose: a purgative mixture was squirted into the anus, using a long pipe and bellows.

QUESTIONS

1   Medieval doctors still believed in the theory of the Four Humours. Did they use it in the same way as doctors in the ancient world?

2   'Medieval medicine did more harm than good.' Do you agree with this statement? Use information from this page in your answer and include:

•   information about preventive medicine

•   information about the treatment of disease.

enquiry

Changes in surgery

One area of medieval medicine in which new discoveries were made was surgery. Surgery was a more practical field than the rest of medicine. It depended less on ideas found in the books of the Greeks and Romans. The constant warfare of the Middle Ages gave surgeons plenty of opportunities to gain experience. In some countries, including Britain, some people combined simple surgery with hairdressing and shaving; they were known as barber-surgeons.

If there is a stone in the bladder, first locate the stone in the following way: have a strong person sit on a bench, his feet on a stool; the patient sits on his lap, legs bound to his neck with a bandage. The surgeon stands in front of the patient and inserts two fingers of his right hand into the anus. The bladder is soft and fleshy so if he finds a hard, firm pellet it is a stone... bring the stone to the neck of the bladder; there at the entrance ... cut lengthwise with a knife and extract the stone.

▲ **SOURCE A** An ambitious medical operation described by Roger Frugardi.

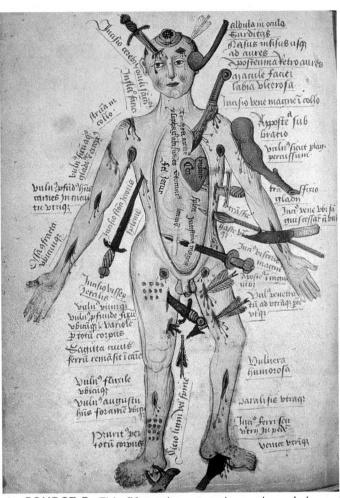

▲ **SOURCE B** This fifteenth century 'wound man' showed surgeons how to deal with different battlefield injuries. It also shows wounds the medieval surgeon felt confident to deal with.

Italy and France were centres for developments in surgery. The top French and Italian surgeons were keen to show that they were well-educated and were more than humble craftsmen. A surgeon called Roger Frugardi of Parma, Italy, wrote a new textbook on surgery in 1180. This textbook was used throughout Europe and was the first of many. Some of Roger's operations were quite ambitious. Take, for example, his approach to the removal of painful bladder stones in Source A.

Ancient writers teach, and almost all modern surgeons follow them, that pus must form in wounds (before the wounds can start to heal). There could be no greater error than this. For pus does nothing but hinder the work of nature, prolong the disease, prevent healing and the closing up of wounds.

▲ **SOURCE C** Theodoric of Lucca, thirteenth century.

In the thirteenth century, two very famous surgeons worked in the Italian city of Lucca; they were Hugh of Lucca and his son, Theodoric of Lucca. They developed new methods of removing arrows from wounds. They used wine on wounds because they had discovered that it reduced the chance of infection. Theodoric wrote a book describing their discoveries. Unusually for the Middle Ages, he openly criticised some of the advice given by Hippocratic writers, particularly on the treatment of wounds.

Other surgeons experimented with primitive forms of **anaesthetic**. It became common for surgeons to give opium-based drugs to patients in order to make them sleepy.

In some universities there were professors of surgery, as well as professors of medicine. These university surgeons pioneered human dissection, which had not taken place earlier in the Middle Ages. From 1340 an annual dissection took place at Montpellier University in France. One of the most famous university surgeons of the Middle Ages was the Frenchman, Guy de Chauliac (1298–1368). He was educated at the universities of Bologna and Montpellier. He wrote a very comprehensive textbook about surgery. As a surgeon, de Chauliac seems to have been very keen to show that he was just as well educated as the university doctors of his day. For this reason his book is full of references to Greek and Roman writers; de Chauliac quoted Galen no fewer than 890 times! De Chauliac had a very ambitious idea of what a good surgeon should be like.

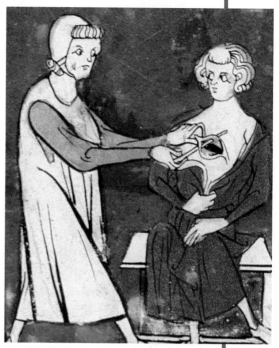

▲ **SOURCE D** This fourteenth-century picture shows a large cut being sutured. The artist has enlarged the wound and the needle to make the technique clear.

KEY WORD

anaesthetic – a pain killer

Four things are necessary for a surgeon: first, he should be very well educated; second, he must have practical expertise; third, he must be honest; and fourth, he should be able to adapt himself to different circumstances. It is essential that a surgeon should not only know the principles of surgery but should also know the theory and practice of medicine in general.

▲ **SOURCE E** Guy de Chauliac, fourteenth century.

QUESTIONS

1 Why do you think medieval surgery was an area in which some progress was made?

2 In what ways was there progress in medieval surgery? In your answer you should mention:

　a operations

　b dealing with pain

　c dealing with infection

　d attitudes towards earlier beliefs.

Concluding your enquiry:
Was progress made in medicine in the Middle Ages?

- list examples of improvements in medicine

- list examples of lack of improvement in medicine

- make your judgement.

Try to write separately about disease and surgery.

enquiry

What was the state of public health in medieval Britain?

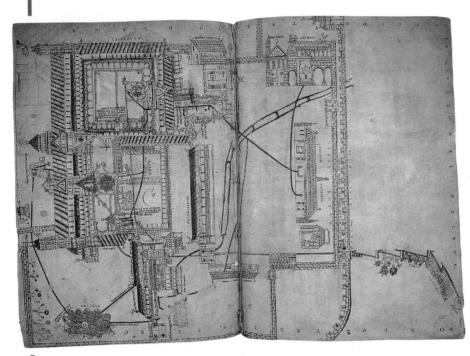

◄ **SOURCE A** Monks and nuns took great care to make sure that they had access to clean water and good sanitation. This plan of 1160 shows the water courses at Canterbury Cathedral Priory. Some of the water channels shown are still in use today.

People sometimes assume that during the Middle Age no one took any interest in hygiene. This is not true. Most wealthy people took some care to keep clean. Childcare books described how people should brush their teeth and use napkins when blowing their noses. Bathing in wooden tubs was common. In the royal household there was always an 'ewerer', or bath-man, whose job it was to provide hot water when the king wanted a bath. King John's bath-man received a payment of 5 pence every time the king had a bath, and we know from royal records that the king usually had a bath once a fortnight. Rich people were also keen to get as far as possible from the stench of human waste. When Henry II built himself a new palace within Dover Castle, he made sure that his bed-room had an 'en-suite' lavatory, or privy, that took the waste far away to a tank at the bottom of the castle keep.

The monks and nuns who lived in monasteries were usually wealthy enough to ensure a good standard of hygiene. New monasteries were located close to supplies of fresh water. In richer monasteries water was piped from building to building. As part of the standard design of a monastery, an elaborate communal lavatory, known as the 'reredorter', was built next to a stream which could carry away the waste. We know from monastic records that monks and nuns washed regularly and had baths five or six times a year.

While the rich took some steps to keep clean, what was life like for poorer people? Most poor people lived in the countryside where there was usually access to clean water and enough space to get rid of waste. We know from records of court cases that when the weather was fine people often bathed in streams and rivers. Court records tell us this because drowning while bathing was a frequent cause of accidental death. In the winter people had baths indoors in tubs. Again there is evidence of this from court records, because scalding bath water sometimes caused fatal accidents.

Health in the towns

By far the greatest public health problems of the Middle Ages were faced by the poor people of the towns. Unlike the rich and the poor of the countryside it was difficult for them to get access to clean water and good quality sanitation. Unlike in the Roman period, the national governments of the Middle Ages did not see public health as their responsibility. Ordinary people did care about hygiene. In London in 1299, a fight broke out when two men criticised a young nobleman for relieving himself in the street. They told him that it was not 'decent' and that he should have used the public lavatory. These public lavatories were often provided by generous rich people when they died and made a will. Dick Whittington, of pantomime fame, left money in his will for a large public lavatory to be built next to the River Thames in London. There were separate sections for men and women, each with toilet seats for 64 people. The waste dropped onto the river bank and was washed away at high tide.

Most town houses had privies, with cess-pits for storing the waste either in back-yards or in cellars. In many cases this meant a dark, smelly pit underneath a wooden toilet seat. Medieval records show children and adults sometimes falling in, on occasion with fatal results. One London man called Richard le Rakiere was sitting on the wooden bench in his privy when the rotten wood gave way. He fell in and was drowned. This is rather ironic because his surname indicates that his job was working as a 'rakier'; these were the people who cleaned out cess-pits for a living.

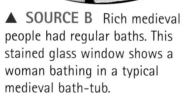

▲ **SOURCE B** Rich medieval people had regular baths. This stained glass window shows a woman bathing in a typical medieval bath-tub.

People who lived in apartments on higher stories of buildings rarely had privies; they had to go down to the ground floor and use a communal lavatory or go out and use a public lavatory. Court records show that sometimes people took the easier option and disposed of their waste out of the window of their apartment. The stench from privies was often commented upon. Privies were typically emptied once every two years.

Town councils and hygiene

Some town councils tried hard to keep the environment clean and healthy. The council of the city of London employed rakiers whose job it was to clean cess-pits, and pick up rubbish and waste. If rich local people failed to pay for public lavatories, this was done by some town councils. Local regulations were introduced ordering trades people, like butchers, to get rid of their waste. Although town councils did try to help public health, they were not as energetic as town councils in some other parts of Europe, particularly in Italy.

QUESTION

Some people think that everyone in the Middle Ages was unhygienic. Imagine that you have been commissioned by BBC Radio to make a programme exploring this issue called 'Were the Middle Ages smelly?' In your script you should mention:

a hygiene and the rich, including royalty and monasteries

b hygiene and the countryside

c towns and hygiene.

Medieval towns

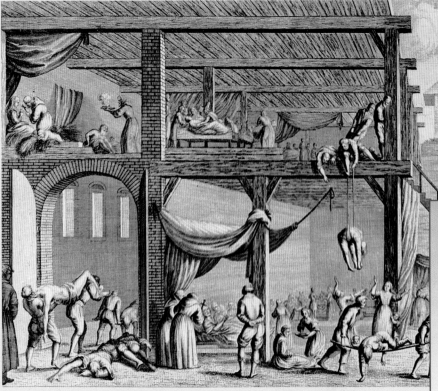

▲ **SOURCE A** A hospital for plague victims in Vienna, 1679.

The city of London went to considerable efforts to keep its streets clean. For the most part, the system seems to have worked well. Although not clean by our standards, the streets that children played in were not as filthy as modern mythology about medieval times would have them seem.

▲ **SOURCE B** Professor Barabara Hanawalt of Minnesota University, writing in *Growing up in Medieval London* (1995).

Maintaining even the most elementary sanitary standards was an enormous problem. In medieval Winchester there is archaeological evidence that there were heaps of refuse in every street and numerous dung-hills, especially near markets, inns and other places where people gathered. Pollution of water supplies was a special problem since they depended heavily upon open streams which were also used for washing clothes (including babies' napkins), for depositing entrails and blood by butchers. More problems were posed by human waste, by privies which flowed into water courses, or those built so close to a neighbour's property that it was invaded by sewage.

▲ **SOURCE C** Edward Miller and John Hatcher, both historians at the University of Cambridge, writing in their book *Medieval England – Towns, Commerce and Crafts* (1995).

Thomas at Wytte and William de Hockele who got together and built latrines which projected out from the walls of the houses on to the lane called Ebbegate. From these latrines human filth falls on to the heads of the passers by and blocks the way through.

▲ **SOURCE D** London Court Records, 1321.

and public health

To the Lord Mayor of London
Order to cause the human faeces and other filth lying in the streets and lanes in the city to be removed with all speed to places far distant ... and to cause the city and suburbs to be cleaned from all odour so that no great cause of mortality may arise from such smells. The King has learned how the city and suburbs are so foul with the filth from out of the houses that the air is infected and the city poisoned to the danger of men.

▲ **SOURCE E** Edward III; an order issued by the king in April 1349.

At the court of Robert Chichele, Lord Mayor of London, it was decided that:
- *the master of Ludgate often puts dung out on to the street and blocks the water flowing into the gutter*
- *the public lavatory at Ludgate is broken and dangerous, and the filth from there is rotting the stone walls.*

▲ **SOURCE F** London Court Records, 1422.

☑ **EXAM TIP**

Make sure you can compare public health in Britain in the Middle Ages with public health in Roman Britain.

The typical borough of the later Middle Ages was not after all such a bad place to live. Throughout the Middle Ages standards of urban cleanliness and hygiene were rising. Town authorities, from the thirteenth century, had concerned themselves with the paving and the cleansing of the streets. There were public latrines in late medieval London, Leicester, Winchester, Hull, Scarborough, Southampton and Exeter. There were supplies of fresh water, brought by pipe or conduit by the town council at London, Exeter, Southampton and Bristol by the fourteenth century.

▲ **SOURCE G** Professor Colin Platt of Southampton University, writing in his book *The Medieval Town* (1976).

QUESTIONS

1   Look at Sources B, C and G These are all modern interpretations. In what ways do they agree about public health in medieval towns?

2   Look at Sources D, E and F. Do they support the idea that medieval towns were successful in providing public health facilities?

3   In what ways do Sources C, D and F show that medieval people did not care about hygiene?

4   What do the visual sources on pages 72, 73 and 74 tell us about whether medieval people cared about hygiene?

5   'Medieval town councils completely failed to provide public health for people.' Using these sources and your background knowledge explain whether you agree with this statement.

You may wish to refer to the following things in your answer:

- the streets
- the removal of sewerage
- funding improvements
- public toilets
- the control of new building
- the control of citizens' behaviour
- clean water
- the passing of laws

The Black Death

Introduction

In October 1347, a fleet of Italian merchant ships docked in the port of Messina. The sailors on board were all dead or dying of a new and terrifying disease. The plague had arrived in western Europe. The first great outbreak of the plague in late medieval Europe is known to history as the Black Death. In the following three years Europe suffered the single greatest medical disaster in its history. One third of the population of Europe died, and in some places the death rate was much higher.

What was the cause of the plague? Although it was not understood at the time, the Black Death was almost certainly an example of bubonic plague. The word 'bubonic' refers to the buboes, or boils, which were a key symptom of the disease. The micro-organism that causes the disease is known by modern scientists as *Yersinia Pestis*. It is carried by rats, and transmitted to humans via fleas. Infected fleas bit nearby humans and spread the killer disease. It was also possible to spread the disease directly from person to person by coughing; this form of the disease is known as pneumonic plague.

Bubonic plague has an **incubation** period of about three days before the symptoms show. Patients get hard painful boils under the armpits, in the groin area and on the neck. Other symptoms include: fever, dark skin blotches, vomiting blood and delirium. Most people died within three to five days of the outbreak of the first symptoms.

People in the Middle Ages did not understand the way micro-organisms caused a disease such as the plague. What explanations for the plague did they have instead? Look at these sources and work out some of the different medieval explanations for the disease.

▲ **SOURCE A** The bubonic plague is spread by a flea which lives on the black rat. Fourteenth-century people had no idea that this was the cause of the disease. How did they explain the Black Death?

KEY WORD

incubation – the period of time between the arrival of micro-organisms in a sick person's body and the first sign of symptoms

QUESTION

Why did people in the Middle Ages not understand what really caused the Black Death?

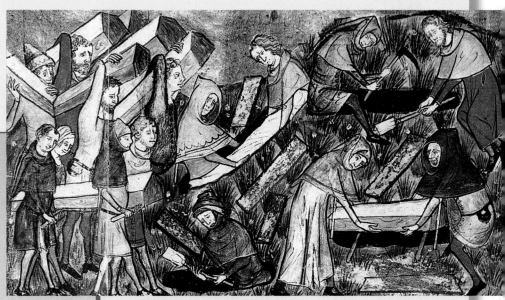

▲ SOURCE B Victims of the Black Death are buried. The disease had a devastating impact on medieval Europe.

The plague came to Strasbourg in the summer of 1349, and about 16,000 people died. The Jews throughout the world were accused of having caused the plague through the poison which they are said to have put into streams and wells. For this reason the Jews were burnt all the way from the Mediterranean to Germany. On Saturday – that was St Valentine's Day – they burnt the Jews of Strasbourg on a wooden platform in the Jewish cemetery. There were about 2,000 of them. Those who wanted to baptize themselves were spared. Many small children were taken out of the fire and baptized against the will of their fathers and mothers. And everything that was owed to the Jews was cancelled, and the Jews had to surrender all the records of money owed to them. All the cash that the Jews possessed was taken and divided among the working-men of the town. The money was indeed the thing that killed the Jews. If they had been poor and if powerful people had not been in debt to them, they would not have been burnt. Thus were the Jews burnt at Strasbourg, and in the same year in all the cities of the Rhineland.

▲ SOURCE C An extract from the chronicle of the Strasbourg historian, Jacob von Königshofen (1346–1420).

Council regulations from the Italian city of Pistoia 1348

I *To stop any contamination presently in the nearby area getting into the bodies of the citizens of Pistoia, no one shall dare to leave the city. And no one can come from outside to the said city of Pistoia on penalty of £50.*

II *No person shall dare to send to the city of Pistoia, any used cloth, either linen or woollen, for use as clothing for men or women or for bedclothes on penalty of £200.*

III *A dead body cannot be removed from the place in which it was found unless first it has been placed in a wooden coffin covered by a lid secured with nails, so that no stench can issue forth from it.*

IV *In order to avoid the foul stench which the bodies of the dead give off every body must by buried in a deep pit.*

▲ SOURCE D Pistoia is 30 kilometres from Florence. These council regulations were introduced in the spring of 1348.

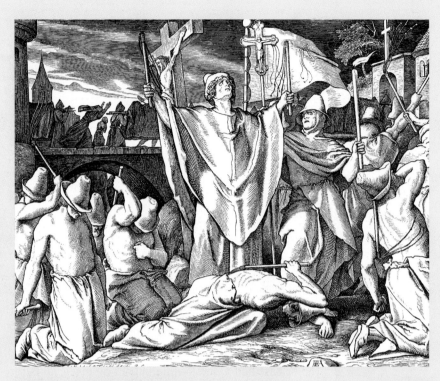

◀ **SOURCE E** A religious procession calls upon God to stop the plague. Flagellants flog themselves to show God that they are sorry for their sins. What did people like this think had caused the disease?

The Scots, hearing of the cruel pestilence in England, imagined that it had come about at the hand of an avenging God, and they said, when they wished to swear, 'by the foul death of England'. Thus believing that a terrible vengeance of God had overtaken the English, they gathered in Selkirk forest with the intention of invading the kingdom of England. There the horrible death overtook the Scots themselves, so that in a short time about 5,000 of them had perished. And as the rest, some strong, some feeble, were preparing to return to their own country, they were surprised by pursuing Englishmen, who killed a great number of them.

▲ **SOURCE F** Henry Knighton, an English monk and historian, writing in the fourteenth century.

It was 1348 when, into the great city of Florence, came the death-dealing plague. As a result of our wickedness, the plague was sent down upon mankind for punishment by the just wrath of God. Nothing could stop its spread. The officers of the city banned sick people from entering. Many processions and other religious services were held begging God to help. Despite these efforts it began to appear in the city in spring 1348. In men and women alike there appeared at the beginning of the sickness, swellings, either on the groin or under the armpits, as big as an apple or an egg. From these two parts of the body the death-bearing plague boils spread quickly to every part of the body. After a while black or fierce red blotches appeared, first on the arms and about the thighs and then spread to every other part of the person. These were a very certain sign of coming death.

▲ **SOURCE G** From *The Decameron* by Boccaccio, an Italian writer who lived through the plague in the city of Florence.

The truth was that there were two causes. The general cause was the close position of the three great planets, Saturn, Jupiter and Mars. This had taken place in 1345 on the 24th March, in the 14th degree of Aquarius. Such a coming together of planets is always a sign of wonderful, terrible or violent things to come. The particular cause of the disease in each person was the state of the body – bad digestion, weakness and blockage, and for this reason people died.

▲ **SOURCE H** Guy de Chauliac, the French surgeon and medical writer.

QUESTIONS

1 How many different explanations for the Black Death can you find in these sources? Which of these explanations are supernatural and which ones involve natural approaches to disease?

2 Which of these sources are useful for historians researching:

   a the symptoms of the plague
   b the action people took to prevent the plague
   c the relationship between Christians and other groups of medieval people
   d the relationship between Scotland and England?

3 These sources do not agree as to what caused the Black Death. Does this mean they are all wrong? Use the sources and your own knowledge in your answer.

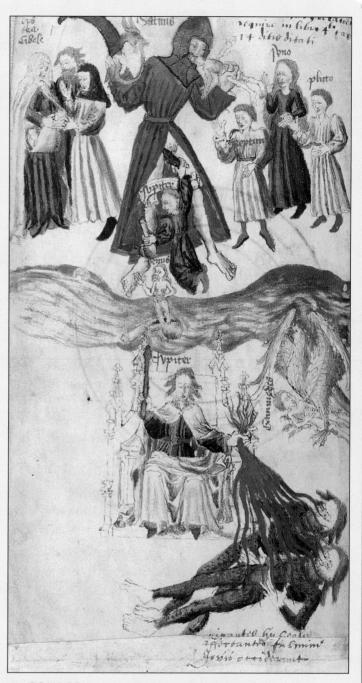

▲ **SOURCE I** A medieval astrological chart shows the coming together of Saturn (shown eating his children) and Jupiter (shown throwing a thunderbolt). This combination of planets was thought to cause disasters.

☑ **EXAM TIP**

If you only use the sources you might agree with the statement in question 3, so make sure you use your *own* knowledge so you can disagree.

review

Was there any progress in medicine during the Middle Ages?

To make sense of medieval medicine, we need to compare it with what went before in the Roman period. In many ways medicine 'regressed' when the Roman Empire in western Europe collapsed and the Middle Ages began:

- Proper training for doctors stopped

- Roman public health systems were abandoned

- Many Greek and Roman medical books were lost.

It is important not to over-estimate the level of regression. Some practical medical knowledge remained in western Europe. High level medical thinking carried on in the eastern Byzantine empire. Above all, the Islamic world rescued much of the work of Greek and Roman medical writers, and developed new medical ideas.

The changes from the Roman to medieval periods demonstrate the importance of **government** and **war**.

The Church's contribution to medieval medicine is complicated. The medieval Church is, therefore, a good example to use when answering a question about the complex impact of religion on medicine. In some ways medieval religion hindered medical knowledge; in some ways it supported medical knowledge. Look at each of the following aspects of medicine. For each one, use your knowledge of the medieval Church to say whether it was a hindrance or a help:

- the keeping of manuscripts in monasteries

- supernatural explanations of disease

- the Church and the hospital system

- the Church's attitude towards scientific research.

Look back at your work on Islamic medicine. What was the contribution of each of these key individuals:

- Rhazes
- Ibn Sina?

The impact of government
After the break up of the Roman Empire, governments became weaker and had much less sense of public health responsibility.
Significantly in the Islamic world there was progress under the rule of the Caliphs of Baghdad, who had a strong government with an interest in science and who were not threatened by war until the thirteenth century.

Progress and regress in medicine

The impact of war
The early Middle Ages was a time of almost constant war; the chaos of the wars hindered medical knowledge.
One exception to this was the field of surgery, where warfare helped progress because it gave surgeons opportunities to treat wounds.

☑ **EXAM TIP**

The Middle Ages are often seen as a period when medicine developed little or even regressed. Make sure you know why this idea is inaccurate.

The level of progress in medieval medicine varied across the different aspects of medicine. Look at each of the following pieces of information. Can you remember any more relevant information from your study of this aspect of medieval medicine? Decide, for each aspect of medicine, whether it indicates progress, regress or stagnation:

The wars of the period gave surgeons opportunities to try new ideas. Textbooks were written that described some new techniques. The Italians, Hugh and Theodoric of Lucca (thirteenth century), criticised Greek and Roman ideas about how wounds healed.

Anatomical knowledge changed little in medieval times. Galen was seen by most doctors as the last word on the subject, so little research took place. Dissection of the human body did not happen for most of the Middle Ages. Some dissection did take place from 1300–1500, but it was used to illustrate Galen's teaching and not for real research.

Medieval Medicine

Was there progress in:

- surgery
- public health
- explanations of disease
- training for doctors
- anatomy?

Roman public health systems collapsed in much of western Europe AD400–600. At the same towns became much smaller, so there was less of a problem with hygiene in crowded towns. There was a growth in town populations after AD1100. Many town councils tried hard to keep the streets clean. Despite their efforts, late-medieval towns were usually dirty, dangerous places for poor people.

Universities were set up across Europe in the years 1200–1500. Many of them had schools of medicine, and for the first time since Roman times there was a high level of training for doctors. While the standard of training for doctors went up, the new universities excluded women healers and would not recognise them as proper doctors.

Explanations of disease changed little during the Middle Ages. Most doctors followed the Greek idea of the Four Humours; people got sick because the humours were out of balance. Belief in the Four Humours led to regular use of blood-letting as a way of trying to prevent disease. As in Ancient Egyptian times, some people saw disease as a supernatural punishment, and prayed to get supernatural cures.

overview

Welcome to the Renaissance

Timeline

- **1492** Christopher Columbus sails to America
- **1517** Martin Luther begins the Reformation; Protestants break away from the Catholic Church
- **1519** The Renaissance artist, Leonardo da Vinci, dies
- **1588** The English defeat the Spanish Armada
- **1609** The telescope is invented
- **1642** The scientist, Galileo, dies

Historians consider that the Middle Ages ended when a number of important new ideas swept through Europe in the fifteenth and sixteenth centuries. The new period that then started is known as the Renaissance, which is a French word meaning 're-birth'. People at the time believed that great progress was being made in many fields because the love of knowledge had been re-born.

What were the key characteristics of the Renaissance?

Artists and sculptors began to think about the human body in a new way. They started showing the body, and other aspects of the natural world, in a realistic way. These **new artistic ideas** first developed in Italy and slowly spread to the rest of Europe.

The Renaissance was an **age of exploration**. New sea routes to Asia, via Africa, were established. In 1492 Christopher Columbus landed in the Caribbean; Europeans had 'discovered' America. Contact with the 'New World' led to the introduction of new plants and products, such as potatoes, tomatoes and tobacco.

There was a massive increase in the communication of knowledge due to the **invention of the printing press**. This was first developed in Germany in the fifteenth century. Before printing, the production of a book was a very time-consuming exercise. Using the new 'moveable type', printers were able to produce millions of books quickly and cheaply.

During the Renaissance there was a **great increase in scientific research**. Copernicus, a sixteenth-century Polish scientist, developed the idea that the earth went round the sun. This undermined Greek and Roman teaching about how the world worked.

During the Renaissance many people challenged the teachings of the Catholic Church. In much of northern Europe there was a 'Reformation', in which new Protestant churches took over from the Catholics. Overall, the period was one in which there was a **reduction in the power of the church**.

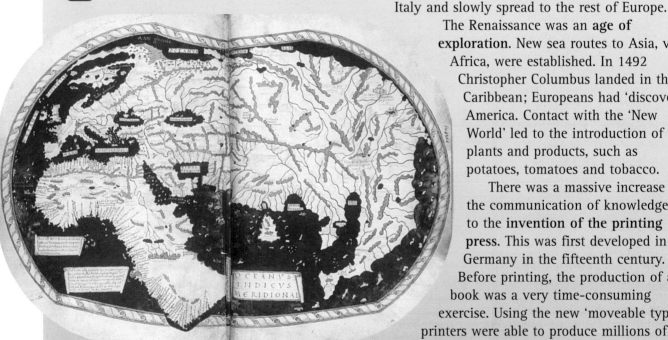

▲ **SOURCE A** This world map of 1489 was made shortly before the discovery of the Americas. The Renaissance was a great period for voyages of discovery.

☑ **EXAM TIP**

Make sure you can work out how each of these key factors might affect medicine.

Leonardo da Vinci

Renaissance man

The spirit of the Renaissance is perhaps best seen in the work of the Italian, Leonardo da Vinci (1452–1519). He was hungry for knowledge in many different fields. We know him best as a great painter, but he was also a brilliant scientist and engineer. In order to produce more realistic paintings and sculpture, Leonardo undertook major research into human anatomy. He carried out dissections and did detailed drawings of the insides of the body. His drawings and notes on anatomy were kept in private notebooks and were never published.

Medieval representations of the body look crude and unrealistic when compared with the art of the Renaissance. It is important to remember that medieval artists had different aims to those of the Renaissance. While Renaissance artists tried to show the body 'as it really is', medieval artists were usually more concerned to produce 'diagrammatic' pictures, simplified pictures that showed the main details. We don't expect a diagram to be realistic in every detail; what matters is that it highlights the most important features.

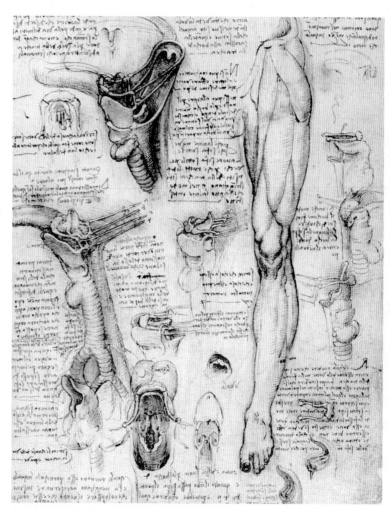

▲ **SOURCE B** There were strong connections between the new art of the Renaissance and medical knowledge. Renaissance artists wanted to know how bodies worked in order to draw them more realistically. Leonardo da Vinci undertook dissections. The anatomical drawings of Leonardo are very different from medieval pictures.

QUESTION

Leonardo da Vinci was not a doctor so why was he important in the history of medicine?

enquiry

What impact did key Renaissance individuals have on medical knowledge?

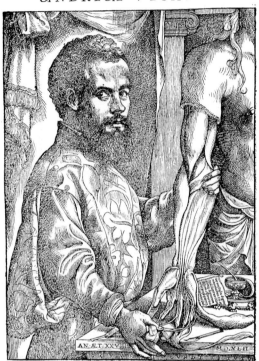

ANDREÆ VESALII.

AN.ÆT.XXVII.

M.D.XLII.

▲ **SOURCE A** Vesalius, as depicted in his great book On the Fabric of the Human Body. This book changed overnight medical knowledge and challenged the teaching of Galen.

Vesalius and the new anatomy

The study of anatomy went through a period of dramatic change in the Renaissance. The single most important figure in this great change is known by his Latin name, Vesalius. His real name was Andreas van Wesele, and he was born in Brussels (in modern Belgium) in 1514. Vesalius was well-connected. His father was pharmacist to Charles V, the German Emperor who also ruled over the territories of modern Belgium and Holland. Vesalius was lucky enough to receive an excellent medical education at the best universities. He studied at the Louvain, Montpellier and Paris universities. As a student he robbed the body of an executed criminal so that he could study it. By the time he became a professor at the great Italian medical university of Padua (in 1537), Vesalius was only 23-years-old.

Vesalius began work in Padua as a faithful follower of Galen. His first publication, in 1538, was a series of anatomical pictures that showed the inside of the body according to the teaching of Galen. This booklet incorrectly described the liver and the heart, reflecting the mistakes made 1400 years before by Galen.

Work at Padua, where there was a long established tradition of dissection, gave Vesalius access to a regular supply of dead bodies for dissection. These were executed criminals. As he carried out more and more dissections he began to have his first doubts about Galen and he concluded that Galen had only carried out dissections on animals. He noticed, for example, that the human lower jaw was different from Galen's description.

☑ EXAM TIP

Note how Vesalius' fame in anatomy depended upon factors unrelated to medicine – the printing press and a good artist!

Vesalius began to write a comprehensive book about human anatomy. This was completed in 1542 and published the following year. It was called *De Humani Corporis Fabrica*, which means 'On the fabric of the human body'. This was the first modern anatomical textbook. It contained 23 full-page anatomical pictures and a further 180 illustrations of different aspects of the inside of the human body. Without the invention of printing such a book would not have been possible. It also depended for its great success on the high quality technical illustrations provided by an artist called Jan van Calcar. Vesalius was the first medical expert to realise the importance of collaboration between doctors and artists. The book was an instant success and Vesalius became famous throughout Europe.

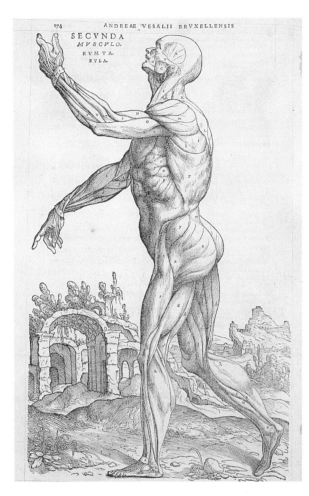

◀ **SOURCE B** With the help of the printing press and a distinguished artist, Vesalius was able to show the internal structure of the human body in a completely new way.

QUESTIONS

1 Briefly describe the life and career of Vesalius based on the following dates – 1514, 1537, 1543, 1564.

2 Look at Source B. Why were drawings like this more useful than earlier drawings of the human body?

3 Vesalius found mistakes in Galen's work. Does this mean Galen should not be seen as important?

4 Why was Vesalius important in the development of medicine?

> ☑ **EXAM TIP**
>
> Make sure you understand that people were important both during their lifetime and later, as their work made the work of others possible.

Several key ideas were to be found in his great book on anatomy:

- Anatomy professors must base their work on dissection and must carry out dissection for themselves.

- The evidence of the eye should be trusted more than the authority of old books.

- Anatomy was the key to further increases in medical knowledge.

- The great doctors of the past made mistakes.

The book corrected several mistakes made by Galen:

- The sternum has three not seven parts.

- The liver does not have five parts or 'lobes'.

- The septum of the heart is not porous.

His thoughts about the septum of the heart were a real breakthrough because they encouraged others to start work on the real answer to how the blood went round the body.

Strangely, Vesalius himself did not continue to publish further researches. Instead he went to work for the rest of his life as personal doctor to the Emperor. He was shipwrecked and drowned in 1564 during a pilgrimage to Jerusalem. Other anatomists followed Vesalius and built on his achievements. His immediate successor at Padua was Realdo Colombo. He proved that blood went from the right to left ventricles via the lungs. Blood was mixed with air in the lungs and changed colour to bright red. In 1551 Gabriele Falloppia went to work at Padua. He researched the workings of the womb and the Falloppian tubes of the womb are still named after him. From 1565 the professor at Padua was a man called Fabricius. His great work was a detailed study of the valves of the veins. Vesalius had been a generalist; his work covered the whole of the human body. Anatomists who followed him, like Falloppia and Fabricius, were specialists who concentrated their research on specific parts of the body.

enquiry

Ambroise Paré and changes in surgery

We seen have seen that surgery was one area of medicine in which some progress was made in the Middle Ages. Further practical improvements in surgery took place during the Renaissance period. The greatest figure in the development of Renaissance surgery was the French man, Ambroise Paré.

Paré was born in 1510. He had a very limited education and could not read Latin, the scientific language of the time. As a boy he was apprentice to a barber. He then became a barber-surgeon at the great Paris hospital of Hôtel Dieu. A turning point in his career came in 1536 when he went as a military surgeon to join the French army as it campaigned in Italy.

◀ **SOURCE C** Ambroise Paré was the greatest surgeon of the Renaissance. He was not well educated and could not understand Latin. He learned much as a military surgeon during wars in Italy.

After this he regularly divided his time between work at the hospital in Paris and military service as a surgeon. His writings on surgery won him considerable fame and, in 1552, he became surgeon to the French king. He died in 1590.

When Paré began work as a military surgeon, the latest thinking on the treatment of gunshot wounds was to be found in a textbook written by an Italian surgeon, Giovanni Vigo (c. 1460–1520). Vigo stated that gunpowder was a form of poison and that gunshot wounds were poisoned. In order to counteract the poison he recommended that they should always be cauterised either with a red-hot iron or with boiling oil. This was both extremely painful and did more harm than good. Paré devised an alternative approach to dealing with these wounds. As we can see from reading Paré's own account of this discovery (Source D), it was, in part, an accident.

I had never seen gunshot wounds before. I had read Jean de Vigo's book on wounds. He says that gunshot wounds must be cauterised with scalding hot oil. This I did at first. After a while I ran out of oil and instead I had to use a dressing of egg yolk, rose oil and turpentine. That night I could not sleep with worry that the wounded would be dead because I had not cauterised them. I got up early to visit them. To my surprise I found those treated with the dressing to be comfortable having rested well. The others, that I had cauterised with boiling oil, were feverish and had great pain. At that moment I decided never again to burn men who were wounded with gunshot.

▲ **SOURCE D** Paré's first encounter with war: Turin 1536.

> **KEY WORD**
>
> cauterise – to burn with a hot iron as a medical treatment

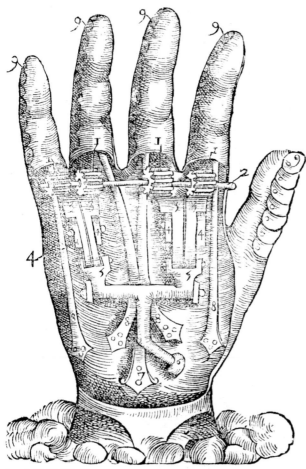

▲ **SOURCE E** Paré tried to help injured soldiers by designing some pioneering false limbs, such as the artificial hands shown here and below.

Paré continued to experiment with more humane ways of treating gunshot wounds. In 1545 he published his findings and criticised Vigo's belief in the need for cauterisation with boiling oil. At first many surgeons rejected his findings. In 1552 an Italian surgeon, Alfonso Ferri published an attack on Paré's approach to the treatment of wounds. Gradually, Paré's more humane approach became accepted as the standard treatment.

Paré's next great contribution to surgical techniques was in the way patients were treated after amputation. The traditional method was simply to cauterise the remaining limb after an amputation with a red-hot iron. Paré developed the use of 'ligatures' instead; this involved tying cut veins and arteries to stop the bleeding. Other surgeons had experimented with ligatures before Paré, but he was the first to give practical guidance as to how it could be done. Paré was keen to share his findings on ligatures and he published his findings in 1552. Paré was a religious man and he considered that he had been inspired by God to make his discoveries in the use of ligatures. In his account of the use of ligatures he wrote, 'This new way was taught me by the special favour of the sacred Deity, for I learnt it not of my masters.' He often said, 'I treated, God cured'.

While the treatment of gunshot wounds and the use of ligatures were Paré's greatest innovations, he took an interest in many other fields of surgery and medicine. He campaigned against the use of worthless 'panaceas'; these were exotic imported drugs that were meant to have curing powers for many ailments. In one extraordinary experiment he showed the king that a drug known as bezoar was useless by deliberately poisoning a man. Bezoar was a stone found inside goats in Persia; when ground up it was supposed to be an antidote for all poisons. The king was curious about this drug and asked Paré, as his surgeon for an opinion. Paré replied that since all poisons were different there could not possibly be a single antidote to all of them. To test his theory a thief awaiting execution was poisoned and then given some bezoar. The thief agreed to the experiment because he was going to be hanged anyway and the king told him that if the drug worked he could go free. The thief died a horribly painful death and the bezoar was shown to be useless.

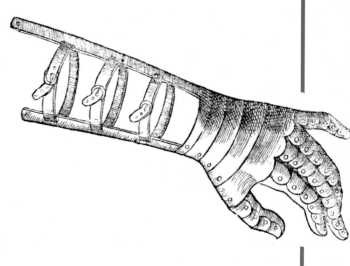

enquiry

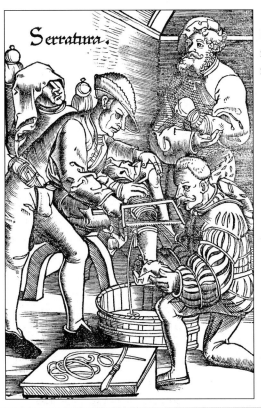

◀ **SOURCE F** The development of ligatures (see page 87) made it much easier to carry out amputations such as this. However, surgery remained painful and the risk of death by infection was still high.

I was about to cut off the thigh of a man of about 40 years of age, and ready to use the saw and cauteries. The sick man began to roar out and tried to run away and was only stopped by my son, who was then very little and was holding the man's thigh. My wife, heavily pregnant, came running out of the next room and grabbed hold of the patient's chest.

▲ **SOURCE F** Fabricius, late sixteenth century.

Later in his career Paré became interested in childbirth. He worked on a technique known as 'podalic version'; this involved turning the baby in the womb so that the baby would not be born feet first.

Throughout his life Paré was keen to get publicity for his findings. He wrote extensively. His books were all in French; this was unusual because most scientific books were written in Latin. In 1575 he produced an edition of collected works that brought together all his earlier key writings. Paré had many critics during his lifetime. Perhaps people were jealous that a poorly educated, practical man should achieve so much fame? There was also snobbery among doctors who did not think that a mere surgeon should have views on medical matters. In 1575 the Paris University School of Medicine criticised him publicly for writing about medicine even though he was not a doctor.

While Paré made some important discoveries we should not overstate the position of surgery after Paré. Surgery remained a painful and dangerous process. Complex internal operations were not possible. Without proper anaesthetics, patients were often in agony during operations. Patients who survived surgery stood a good chance of dying from infection. A grim picture of surgery in the late sixteenth century comes from an account by the Italian surgeon and anatomist, Fabricius (Source G).

QUESTIONS

1 How did Paré change the way that surgeons treated gunshot wounds? What part did war and chance play in his great discovery?

2 How did Paré's use of the ligature change the way amputations took place?

3 How did Paré prove that bezoar was worthless?

4 What problems continued to face surgeons after the death of Paré?

☑ **EXAM TIP**

Paré is another example of how new ideas were often opposed. Make sure you understand why.

Paracelsus and a new approach to disease

One of the most controversial figures of the medical Renaissance was a Swiss scientist known as Paracelsus (1493–1541). He was born Philippus Aureolus Theophrastus Bombastus von Hohenheim. He changed to Paracelsus (meaning 'greater than Celsus') to show that he considered himself to be a better doctor than Celsus, a famous doctor of Roman times.

Paracelsus had some ideas that were entirely different to the teachings of Galen and Hippocrates. He rejected the idea that disease was caused by an imbalance of the Four Humours. Instead, he said that disease resulted from problems with chemicals inside the body. Since the cause of disease was chemical, treatments should also be chemical. He experimented with the use of chemicals to make new medicines. His basic ingredients were salt, sulphur and mercury.

In 1526, he became town doctor and professor of medicine in the Swiss city of Basel. He showed his contempt for traditional university medicine by refusing to wear academic robes and lecture in Latin. Instead he gave his talks to students in German, the language of the ordinary people. In 1527, he publicly burnt many of the works of Galen and Ibn Sina's 'Canon', which had been the standard university textbook of the late Middle Ages.

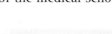

▲ **SOURCE G** Paracelsus: this Swiss doctor strongly rejected the authority of Roman and Greek writers on medicine. In this picture we see him carrying out an operation for the removal of gall stones. He also developed new chemical treatments for illnesses.

Paracelsus seems in many ways a modern figure: he rejected traditional authority and investigated the use of chemical medicines. Not all of his ideas were scientific in modern terms. Paracelsus was a very religious man who believed that God had given people secret messages about how the world worked. He believed in the idea of 'signatures'. Nature identified plants with curing powers. The orchid was shaped like a testicle to show that it could be used for the treatment of sexually transmitted diseases. The plant 'eyebright' (*Euphrasia officianalis*) looked like a blue eye to show that it could be used for the treatment of eye complaints.

The impact of Paracelsus was limited during his own lifetime. Few of his medical writings were published before he died. After his death a small number of followers continued his work, and explored further the use of chemical treatments for disease. Paracelsus was ignored by the leading universities of Europe who saw him as a crank and eccentric. The teachings of Galen remained unchallenged in most of the medical schools in European universities.

> *I tell you, one hair on my neck knows more than all the old authors, and my shoe-buckles contain more wisdom than Galen.*

▲ **SOURCE I** Paracelsus, early sixteenth century.

QUESTIONS

1 What new approach to the nature of disease did Paracelsus develop?

2 What did Paracelsus think of old medical authorities like Galen?

3 Why is it wrong to think of Paracelsus as a completely modern scientist?

4 Did Paracelsus make a big difference to the way most doctors did their work?

enquiry

William Harvey and the circulation of the blood

While Vesalius improved anatomy (the understanding of the inside of the body), he did little work on physiology (how the body works). The Renaissance individual who did the most to improve knowledge of physiology was the English doctor, William Harvey (1578–1657). Harvey showed conclusively that blood circulates around the body: the blood is pumped away from the heart through the arteries and returns to the heart via the veins. Not only was this an important discovery, but the way Harvey approached the problem showed how new knowledge about the body could be gained through experimentation and careful observation.

Before Harvey's work, thinking about the heart was still dominated by the ideas of Galen. The two ventricles of the heart are divided by a wall known as the septum. Galen had stated that the blood must move from one ventricle to the other through invisible minute openings or pores. As the blood went from the heart it was, according to Galen, 'burnt up' or absorbed by the body.

In 1628 Harvey published a book on the circulation of blood. It begins with an attack on Galen's ideas. Galen had said that veins carried both blood and air. Harvey pointed out that when examined, veins only ever contained blood. Harvey totally rejected the idea of the invisible pores that link together the ventricles: 'By Hercules, there ARE no such porosities, and they cannot be demonstrated.'

Harvey's ideas

In the second half of his book Harvey argued that blood circulates around the body. He used information from experiments to show how much blood was pumped by the heart and that it could not be simply absorbed by the body. The blood must go round and round the body otherwise the body would not be able to cope with the huge amount of blood pumped out by the heart. Harvey used information from simple experiments on the

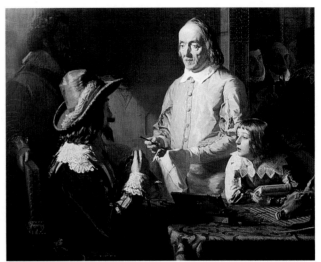

▲ **SOURCE A** A nineteenth-century painting shows Harvey explaining the circulation of the blood to his patron, King Charles I. How did other people react to his discovery?

veins and arteries of the arm to show that blood flowed down the arteries and returned up the veins. Although he could not see them, Harvey established that there must be tiny channels that connected the artery system to the vein system so that circulation could take place. His study of the valves of the veins and the arteries confirmed his view of the different functions of these blood vessels.

Look at Source B, showing pictures from Harvey's book. They show how a tight tie, or ligature, round the arm stops blood flowing out of the arm and also makes the veins and valves stand out so that they can be clearly seen. In Figure 2 Harvey put his finger just above a valve and strokes the blood upwards and out beyond the next valve. The empty vein becomes invisible. In Figure 3 he tries to force blood backwards down the vein. This does not work because the valve only allows blood to flow one way, up the arm. In this way Harvey showed that the veins only existed to take blood back to the heart.

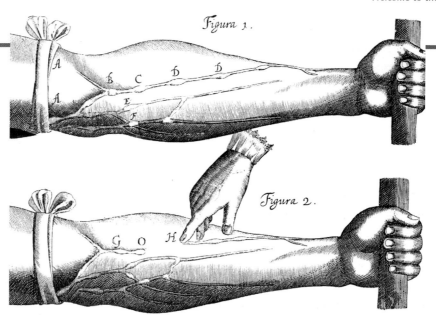

Figura 1.

Figura 2.

▲ **SOURCE B** These pictures are the only illustrations in Harvey's book.

Harvey's explanation of his theory was brilliant. This did not mean that people accepted his new ideas. Quite the contrary, there was a huge controversy about his book and many doctors flatly refused to accept that Harvey was right and Galen was wrong.

Doctors and other scientists found it very difficult to come to terms with Harvey's discovery. Some responded by simply ignoring Harvey. Others vigorously attacked Harvey. English medical textbooks continued to give Galen's account until 1651. Harvey received a very hostile reception from Paris University. It was not until 1673 that medical lectures in Paris began to teach Harvey's ideas rather than Galen's.

Place a ligature on the arm of some poor wretch. Torture him to please Harvey and see what happens. The terrible pain attracts blood into his veins. Is it any wonder they appear swollen?

▲ **SOURCE D** An Italian doctor, Emilius Parisanus, completely rejected Harvey's ideas and made fun of his experimental methods in a book published in 1635.

QUESTIONS

1 a How did Galen explain the way the heart worked?

   b What mistake did Galen make?

2 How did Harvey show that the blood circulated round the body?

3 Source B shows the only picture in the whole of Harvey's book. Explain in your own words what this picture shows and why it was so important to Harvey.

4 a How did people react to Harvey's discovery?

   b Why do you think that many people opposed his new ideas?

Concluding your enquiry:

What impact did key Renaissance individuals have on medical knowledge?

- Write down all the discoveries made by the four individuals featured in this enquiry.
- Consider the importance of opposition to their work.
- Make your decision.

To take your understanding even further think about how some of their discoveries paved the way for further developments.

enquiry

What was the impact of the plague on seventeenth-century Britain?

A FORM
OF
COMMON PRAYER,
TOGETHER
With an Order of Fasting,
FOR THE
Averting of Gods heavy Visitation
Upon many places of this Realm.
THE
FAST
To be observ'd within the Cities of *London* and
Westminster, and places adjacent,
On Wednesday the Twelfth of this instant July;
And both there, and in all parts of this Realm,
On the First Wednesday in every Moneth:
AND THE
PRAYERS
To be Read
On Wednesday in every *Week*,
During this *Visitation.*
Set forth by His Majesties Authority.

LONDON,
Printed by *John Bill* and *Christopher Barker*,
Printers to the Kings most Excellent Majesty, 1665.

▲ **SOURCE A** Regulations ordering people to pray and fast (stop eating) to persuade God to stop the plague. Did most people explain the plague in supernatural terms?

The plague, that first devastated Britain in 1348, continued to cause widespread death and misery for the next 300 years. Major epidemics broke out on average once every 15 or 20 years. The last great outbreak of the plague in Britain took place in 1665. It is known as the Great Plague. The death toll in London was particularly high and the horror of the summer of 1665 was captured in the diary of Samuel Pepys, a wealthy Londoner (Source B).

June 7 1665
This day I did in Drury Lane see two or three houses marked with a red cross upon the doors, and 'Lord have mercy upon us' writ there. This was a sad sight to me, being the first of the kind, to my remembrance, I ever saw. I was forced to buy some roll-tobacco to smell and chew, which took away my apprehension.

September 14 1665
One of my own water-men that carried me daily, fell sick as soon as he had landed on Friday morning and is now dead of the plague. Both my servants, Hewer and Edwards have lost their fathers of the plague this week.

▲ **SOURCE B** From *The Diary of Samuel Pepys.*

☑ EXAM TIP

Use this enquiry into the Great Plague to show the continuity of supernatural approaches to disease. Make sure you can comparé reactions to the Black Death to those of the Great Plague.

What is the cause that this pestilence is so great in one part of the land but not in another? Only that it pleaseth the Lord in wisdom to defend some but not the rest. Therefore let us believe that in these dangerous times God must be our only defence.

▲ **SOURCE C** Nicholas Bownd, *Medicines for the Plague* (1604).

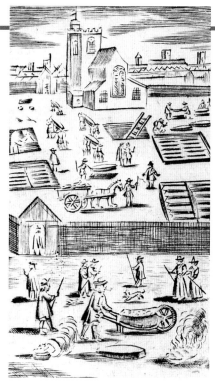

▲ **SOURCE D** Plague victims are buried at night in a very well organised way. What other precautions did the London authorities take to stop the plague?

While many people stressed religious causes, most educated people in the seventeenth century thought that there were rational causes of the plague, and so practical steps could be taken to reduce the spread of the disease. The following source is an extract from a clergyman's explanation of the disease. It is interesting that he makes no reference to God as the cause:

> It is as clear as the sun that the recent increase of the pestilence came by the carelessness of the people, and their greediness in receiving infected goods into their houses.

▲ **SOURCE E** William Laud, to Thomas Wentworth, 1637.

Attempts to control the Plague in London: government as a factor in the development of medicine

The centre of London was the responsibility of the council of the City of London, headed by the Lord Mayor. In 1665 the City council and the Lord Mayor took practical steps to control the disease:

Regulations of the City of London Council 1665

- Examiners and searchers should be appointed, whose job it is to identify houses where the plague has struck and board the houses up to stop the spread of the infection.

- An infected house should be shut up for a month, and no one allowed to leave unless they go to a special plague hospital called a pest-house. Boarded up houses should be marked with a large cross and the words 'Lord have mercy on us'.

- Watchmen should be appointed to guard the houses and make sure that no one escapes.

- People inside infected houses should be supplied with essential food by the council if they are too poor to pay for their own food.

- The dead are only to be buried at night.

- Stray dogs are to be killed by council dog-killers. No other animals should be kept in the City.

How much credit can the City of London take for these plague regulations? Most historians of public health would answer 'not much'. The truth is that the national government had been calling for local authorities to take action along these lines for over a century. It was only in 1665 that local councils, such as the City of London, finally agreed to take vigorous steps to limit the plague. From a British perspective most local councils were unwilling to take responsibility for plague prevention throughout the sixteenth and early seventeenth centuries. Local and national governments in much of continental Europe were much more active. In comparison with the sluggish response in Britain, the governments of the different Italian states were particularly energetic in their treatment of the plague. Isolation hospitals for plague victims were called 'lazarettos'. Hospitals of this kind were built in the Italian states of Venice and Milan by the fifteenth century. In Britain, by contrast, isolation hospitals only became common in the seventeenth century.

enquiry

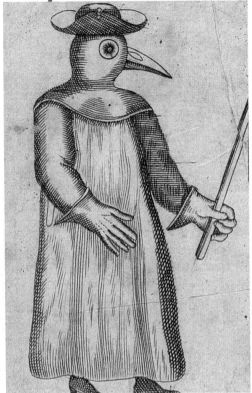

▲ **SOURCE F** Most ideas about treating the plague came from France and Italy. This Italian picture shows the protective clothing that should be worn by those who came into contact with plague victims.

Italians and plague prevention

The Italian approach to plague prevention had a number of strands:

- people suspected of the disease were 'quarantined' – kept out of contact with rest of the population until it was clear that they were free of disease

- travellers were only allowed to enter places if they had a certificate from a doctor stating that they were free from infection

- goods and clothes of infected people were destroyed

- towns had a board of health to keep a check on public health.

Plague in Tudor England

These steps were common practice in Italy in 1500 but only became standard in Britain in the seventeenth century. Early sixteenth century Italian writers warned that England was a dangerous country to visit because it had no effective anti-plague regulations. The Tudor government was aware of this and took some steps put the situation right. The first significant measure came in 1518 when Henry VIII announced that infected houses in London should be identified with bundles of straw hung out of windows for forty days. Those who lived within infected houses should carry a white stick when walking outside their houses. This proclamation was largely ignored and the council of the City of London was reluctant to get involved in public health matters because of the cost. Some members of the city council also thought that the recommended measures were a waste of time because the plague was spread through poisonous air, and nothing practical could be done to stop it.

We wish such of you as have travelled in outward parts [foreign lands] to set forth such devices [measures] as you have seen there observed. So as we may have among us as charitable [caring] a mind for preservation [keeping alive] of our neighbours, as they have.

▲ **SOURCE G** Privy Council order to the City of London, 1543.

In 1543 the royal government urged the City of London Council to take public health more seriously. In particular, the government called upon the council to copy continental public health measures, such as those used in Italy.

These warnings and criticisms did little good. In 1564 the government accused the London authorities of 'great negligence and remiss slackness.' A few other councils, in other parts of the country, took public health more seriously. York council was unusually active in the fight against plague infection. It said, as early as 1536,

that strangers should have certificates of health before entering during an epidemic. This practice did not spread to most towns in England until the mid-seventeenth century.

In 1578, the government gave recommendations as to how local councils should act in time of plague. These regulations put into practice very slowly by local councils. For many years the London City authorities refused to follow these recommendations because they would be too expensive. The action taken by the Lord Mayor of London in 1665 was a late acceptance of these regulations.

The Great Fire and the Great Plague: a question of interpretation

The Great Plague of 1665 was the final epidemic in Britain of the bubonic plague. Many books still claim that London was freed of the curse of the plague because a year later, in 1666, the Great Fire of London destroyed much of the city and 'cleansed' it of the plague. Is this a convincing explanation as to why the plague did not return? Think about the following aspects of the story of the Plague and the Great Fire of London:

- The areas most badly affected by the plague were the suburbs where the poorest people lived.

- The area devastated by the Great Fire was the centre of the city where many of the richest people lived, many of the suburbs were untouched.

- The plague struck many British towns in 1665 and then failed to return. London was the only city to be damaged by the Great Fire.

You have probably concluded that that the idea of the Great Fire 'purifying' the city of London is not at all convincing. If this interpretation will not do, how else can we explain that fact that the plague did not return?

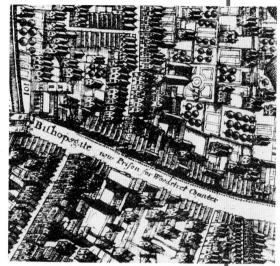

▲ **SOURCE H** The crowded streets of Bishopsgate in London. Did the plague disappear from these streets because of the Great Fire of London?

Historians' ideas

One historian, Paul Slack, has looked in detail at this question. He noticed that the plague still broke out in other parts of the world after 1665, but did not reach north-west Europe. In 1770, for example, Moscow was devastated by the plague. Clearly, the plague was still very dangerous. His view is that the plague did not recur in Britain because neighbouring countries became stricter and stricter in their quarantine rules at ports. In other words, the national and local governments in Britain can take almost no credit for this progress. It was public health measures by authorities in places like France and the Netherlands that meant that after 1665 the plague came nowhere near Britain.

QUESTIONS

1 Explain in your own words the practical steps taken by the London city council during the Great Plague of 1665.

2 What explanations did people have for the plague in Britain in the seventeenth century?

3 In what ways did Italian town councils provide better care for public health long before British town councils?

4 Do you agree with the view that the plague died out in Britain because of the impact of the Great Fire of London? Explain your answer.

5 Between the Black Death and the Great Plague was there much progress in people's ideas about disease?

Concluding your enquiry:

What was the impact of the plague in seventeenth-century Britain?

- Consider the number of casualties, the change to people's lives and the response of government.

- Use this enquiry to show the importance of government as a factor in medicine.

enquiry

> How far did the Renaissance bring about changes in medical treatments?

The impact of the discoveries

What difference did the discoveries of the Renaissance make to the way patients were treated? One of the great figures of the Renaissance, William Harvey, was a practising doctor. Did his discovery of the circulation of blood change the way he treated disease? In a series of lectures to medical students, he described his approach to blood letting:

I would not have it thought that I hold all blood-letting in discredit, as dangerous and injurious, or that I believe with the vulgar [ordinary people] that as blood is lost life is shortened. Daily experience satisfies us that blood letting has a most salutary [healthy] effect in many diseases, and is indeed the foremost of the remedial means [ways of medical treatment]. Vitiated states and plethora of blood are causes of a whole host of diseases. The timely evacuation of a certain quantity of blood frequently delivers patients from very dangerous diseases. This nature teaches, for copious discharges from the nostrils, from hemorrhoids, and in the form of menstrual flux, often deliver us from many diseases.

▲ **SOURCE A** William Harvey, Lumleian lectures (1616–1628).

The health and hygiene of the king of France

French archaeologists have given us information about the health of Louis XIV and his courtiers. Louis became king of France at the age of five in 1643 and reigned for 72 years until his death in 1715. He was the most powerful man in the world. Despite this he seems to have had a number of medical problems. Archaeologists have recently excavated the latrines at the site of a house he used for hunting at Marly-le-Roi, near Paris. In the

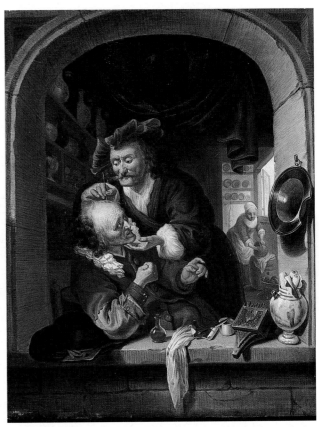

▲ **SOURCE B** A seventeenth-century Dutch painting shows a barber surgeon operating on a man's head. Although it took place at the end of the Renaissance, a scene like this was little different from surgery in the Middle Ages.

remains of human waste they have found evidence that two different parasites were very common. The presence of these internal parasites is evidence of poor hygiene. Almost certainly Louis and his courtiers did not wash their hands properly after going to the lavatory! The archaeologists have also found the eggs of tapeworms. This was almost certainly caused by the consumption of undercoooked meat. Rarely grilled meat was fashionable among the rich in the seventeenth century. Poorer people ate relatively little meat and boiled what little they had, so killing the tapeworms.

The deathbed of Charles II

Historians have available to them a summary of the treatment of Charles II, based on the notes of one of his doctors, Sir Charles Scarburgh.

February 2: The king is taken ill. He felt some unusual disturbance in his brain, followed by loss of speech and convulsions. Two of his doctors are close by. They immediately recommend blood-letting. Sixteen ounces of blood is taken from a vein in his right arm. Messengers are sent urgently summoning his other doctors. Eventually a team of twelve assemble. They meet and decide to take another 8 ounces of blood by placing cupping glasses on his shoulders. They also clear his stomach with an emetic, and give him laxative pills and an enema to empty his bowels. His head is shaved and burnt to make blisters.

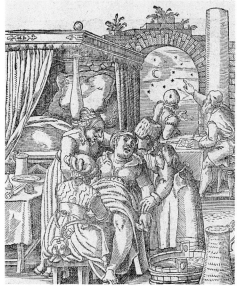

▲ SOURCE C The birth of a baby in the late Renaissance. While female midwives tend to the mother and baby, male astrologers try to predict the baby's future.

February 3: The king takes laxatives continuously. At noon the doctors open the jugular veins and remove ten ounces of blood.

February 4: Laxatives continue to be used. The doctors are becoming desperate and they prescribe a medicine based on ground up human skull.

February 5: The king is given a medicine based on the bark of a Peruvian tree.

February 6: Doctors continue to administer Peruvian bark. They give him a medicine including bezoar: this is a ground up stone from the stomach of an Iranian goat. The king dies.

> ☑ **EXAM TIP**
>
> Make sure you understand how the Renaissance changes gave people ideas to develop later.

QUESTIONS

1. Throughout the Middle Ages, doctors used blood letting to treat patients. Did William Harvey change this treatment because of his discoveries?

2. What does archaeological evidence tell us about the health and hygiene of King Louis XIV and his courtiers?

3. What can we learn from the treatment of Charles II about the standard of medical care at the end of the Renaissance?

Concluding your enquiry:

How far did the Renaissance bring about changes in medical treatments?

- Summarise the ways in which treatments got better in the Renaissance, such as the work of Paré

- Summarise the way that some discoveries had little immediate impact on treatment, such as the work of Vesalius and Harvey

- Summarise some of the problems that remained at the end of the Renaissance

- Balance the changes with the continuities (things that stayed the same).

review

> ## How far were key individuals able to change medicine during the Renaissance?

The Renaissance period is good for considering how individuals can make a difference to medical knowledge because the developments of the period are closely connected with a few key individuals. While these individuals made an important contribution to medicine, their work was made possible by a number of other factors.

Look at the descriptions of Paracelsus, Vesalius, Paré and Harvey. Summarise in your own words how and why they changed accepted ideas.

Medicine at the end of the Renaissance

Although each of the four individuals had expanded medical understanding, many problems remained at the end of the period:

- Doctors did not understand the way micro-organisms cause disease. Although most doctors rejected, for example, supernatural explanations of the bubonic plague, they did not understand the real causes.

- Medical treatment got little better, despite the discoveries of the Renaissance. The work of men like Vesalius and Harvey made no practical difference to the way sick people were treated. The painful death of Charles II, King of England, illustrates this; he was given many painful and worthless treatments before he died.

- Surgery, despite the advances of Paré, remained very limited because of the problems of pain, infection and blood loss. Complex internal operations were impossible.

Paracelsus and a new approach to disease

This Swiss medical writer did not believe in the Four Humours. Instead he explained disease in terms of the chemistry of the body, and called for the use of chemical drugs in medical treatment. He gave his lectures in German, rather than Latin and burnt the works of Galen.

Vesalius and the new anatomy

Appointed at the age of 23 as professor of anatomy at Padua, Vesalius carried out many dissections. He published a remarkable book in 1543: 'On the Fabric of the Human Body'. This book was illustrated with high quality pictures of the inside of the human body. Vesalius showed that Galen had made a number of mistakes in anatomy because he did not use humans for his dissections.

Paré and improvements to surgery

The French surgeon, Ambroise Paré, changed the way battlefield surgery was carried out. Instead of treating gunshot wounds with boiling oil, he developed a new, less painful and more effective dressing of egg yoke and turpentine. This was in part accidental because on one occasion Paré ran out of boiling oil. Paré also showed how cut arteries and veins could be tied in a ligature rather than cauterised. This made amputation much more humane. Paré published his findings in books printed in French rather than Latin. He also proved that many exotic drugs that were supposed to cure everything were, in fact, worthless.

Harvey and the circulation of the blood

William Harvey was an English doctor. He studied at Padua University. Harvey proved that the blood circulated round the body; it was carried away from the heart by arteries and returned to the heart by veins. He disproved Galen's idea that blood moved through invisible 'pores' between the two ventricles of the heart. Harvey's book on the circulation of the blood was published in 1628 and caused a sensation throughout Europe.

overview

Welcome to the Enlightenment and Industrialisation

Timeline

The Enlightenment

The period from the end of the seventeenth century to the end of the eighteenth century in western Europe was called the age of Enlightenment. Leading thinkers believed that 'reason' (that is logical, clear thinking) would create a better future for mankind. Blind obedience to rulers, churches and ideas that were shown to be wrong should be overthrown. There was a belief that progress in science and technology would lead to an ideal existence and, in medicine, the eventual conquest of all disease. The new way of thinking about the world and mankind led to some dramatic changes. Look on the timeline to see them.

Industrialisation

One of the great changes of the eighteenth century was the introduction of factories and the growth of industrial towns. In the nineteenth century industry was the social and wealth base of European countries and the USA. At the same time many scientific discoveries were being made and science was becoming systematic. Science, wealth and industry combined to increase the pace of change. Medicine benefited from these changes. But there was a price to pay. Industrial towns were overcrowded and became places of ill health. Industrialisation meant riches for some but also squalid poverty for others. However, the period of industrialisation saw some of the most important, fundamental discoveries in the development of medicine. The nineteenth century, the time of industrialisation, is also called the time of the medical revolution.

The nature of the Enlightenment

In the eighteenth century the scientific method of research, observation and experiment, begun by Galileo, became accepted. This led to medicine being based upon scientific knowledge. Doctors began to work in a way that we would recognise today. Increased awareness of the sufferings of the poor and the sick led to the foundation of many of the great London teaching hospitals.

The outstanding doctor of the Enlightenment was Herman Boerhaave from Holland. In 1701 he became professor of medicine at the University of Leyden. He taught his students that their place was at the patient's bedside. Theories should take second place to practical observation and the patient's cure.

Doctors should keep notes and post mortems should investigate the cause of death if the patient died. Pathology, the study of the nature of disease and the changes it causes, became a major tool for doctors. Boerhaave's methods inspired large numbers of students from many countries. They took them back to their own countries after their studies and his ideas became the foundation for medical practice in Europe and North America. One of Boerhaave's students was Alexander Monro who established Edinburgh as a major teaching centre for physicians. As we shall see, an Edinburgh-based surgeon, James Simpson, was to have an important influence on the development of medicine (pages 124–25). As well as improved methods for doctors, the Enlightenment also saw other medical advances. William Withering (1741-99) investigated herbal cures and found that foxglove was an effective treatment for heart problems. James Lind discovered that drinking lime juice eliminated the killer disease scurvy on long sea voyages. However, the Enlightenment was also a golden age for 'quack' doctors (see Source A) peddling bizarre and useless remedies. For example, in Britain, James Graham had a 'temple of health' where patients were supposed to be cured by watching dancing girls and receiving mild electric shocks.

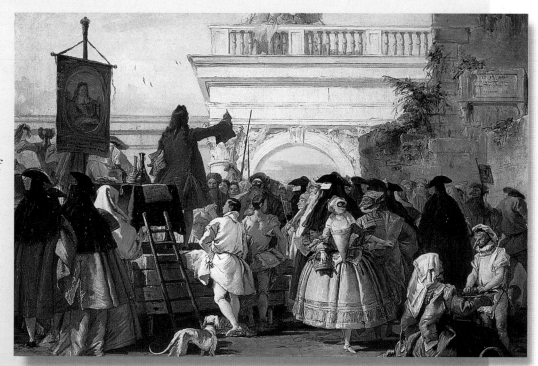

▲ SOURCE A *The Quack Doctor.* An eighteenth-century painting by Tiepolo. The quack persuades some of the crowd to buy his 'medicine' before quickly moving on.

enquiry

Why were new hospitals set up in the eighteenth century?

Medical societies

The new interest in science in the late seventeenth and eighteenth century encouraged the sharing of new ideas. Many people involved in medicine joined the Royal Society. This had been set up in 1662 to encourage new scientific discoveries, but the changes did not end there. In 1732 a medical society was set up in Edinburgh, Scotland. This idea spread and during the eighteenth century a number of different groups were set up in London, where new ideas about medicine could be discussed. These groups, known as societies, provided the only extra training for surgeons and apothecaries who were already involved in looking after the sick. Physicians did have other meetings run by the College of Physicians and there was often rivalry between these groups. The apothecaries said physicians had no interest in treating poor, sick people. Physicians were often jealous of the way people relied on the apothecaries.

New London hospitals

At around the same time many new hospitals were set up in London: Westminster Hospital (1719), Guy's (1721), St George's (1733), The London (1740), The Middlesex (1745). A typical one was Guy's Hospital, which was paid for by Thomas Guy, a rich printer and bookseller. He was one of a number of wealthy people who believed that they should use their money to try to improve the lives of poor and sick people. Many of these rich people were influenced by the Christian belief that the rich should help the poor and that through the development of new ideas, science could improve life. Many rich people hoped that, as a result of their help, the poor would be encouraged to live cleaner and more disciplined lives. The rich believed they were helping to put an end to violent and dangerous behaviour in cities. The poor would be grateful to God and to their rich neighbours.

Reasons for these changes

A number of events combined to bring about these changes in the eighteenth century:

- new ideas from the Enlightenment

- peace in Britain improved the economy and brought more wealth to some people

- richer, better educated people believed God had given them responsibility to improve the lives of the poor

- many existing hospitals were old and needed replacing

- physicians hoped that new hospitals would help them become more powerful than the apothecaries

- growth in medical societies meant there were more people interested in exploring new ways of treating the sick

The sick must acknowledge the goodness of God in providing so comfortable a situation, care, medicine and skill, while under the afflicting hand of God. They must behave soberly and religiously as Christians.

▲ SOURCE A Eighteenth-century rules of Guy's Hospital.

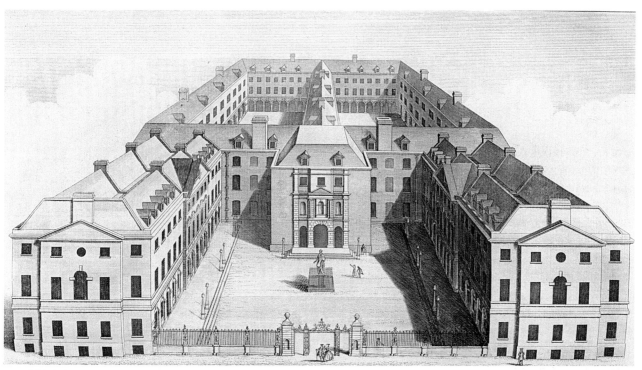

▲ SOURCE B Guy's Hospital, 1734.

Desiring to improve medicine and other sciences and convinced of the great advantages coming from free communication of observations and opinions, we have desired to set up this association.

▲ SOURCE C The aims of the Guy's Hospital Physical Society, 1771.

QUESTIONS

1   What does Source A tell you about Thomas Guy's reasons for setting up Guy's Hospital?

2   How does Source C help explain why it was easier to set up hospitals in the eighteenth century than it had been before?

Concluding your enquiry:
Why were new hospitals set up? Construct a spidergram with as many reasons as you can find from the information in this section.

enquiry

Why were British industrial towns so unhealthy?

During the Industrial nineteenth century many British towns grew immensely in size. For example, in 1800 there were only six towns in Britain with a population of more than 70,000. This is not very large at all by twenty-first-century standards. By 1900 there were 45 places with populations of this size. By 1851, for the first time in British history, there were about as many people living in towns as in the countryside. By 1901 80% of the British population lived in towns, or cities.

This huge growth in urban population had a great impact on the health of the people living in towns and cities. This was especially true of the poorer working class populations.

How did the growth of towns affect health?

The most obvious evidence of the unhealthiness of urban life can be found in the average age of death of town dwellers. In 1842 the average age of death in Manchester was:

- Working Class, 17 years old
- Middle Class, 20 years old
- Upper Class, 38 years old

For working and middle class people this 'life expectancy' was half that of people living in the countryside. Even for upper class people, life in the countryside was healthier, with a life expectancy of about 52 years there.

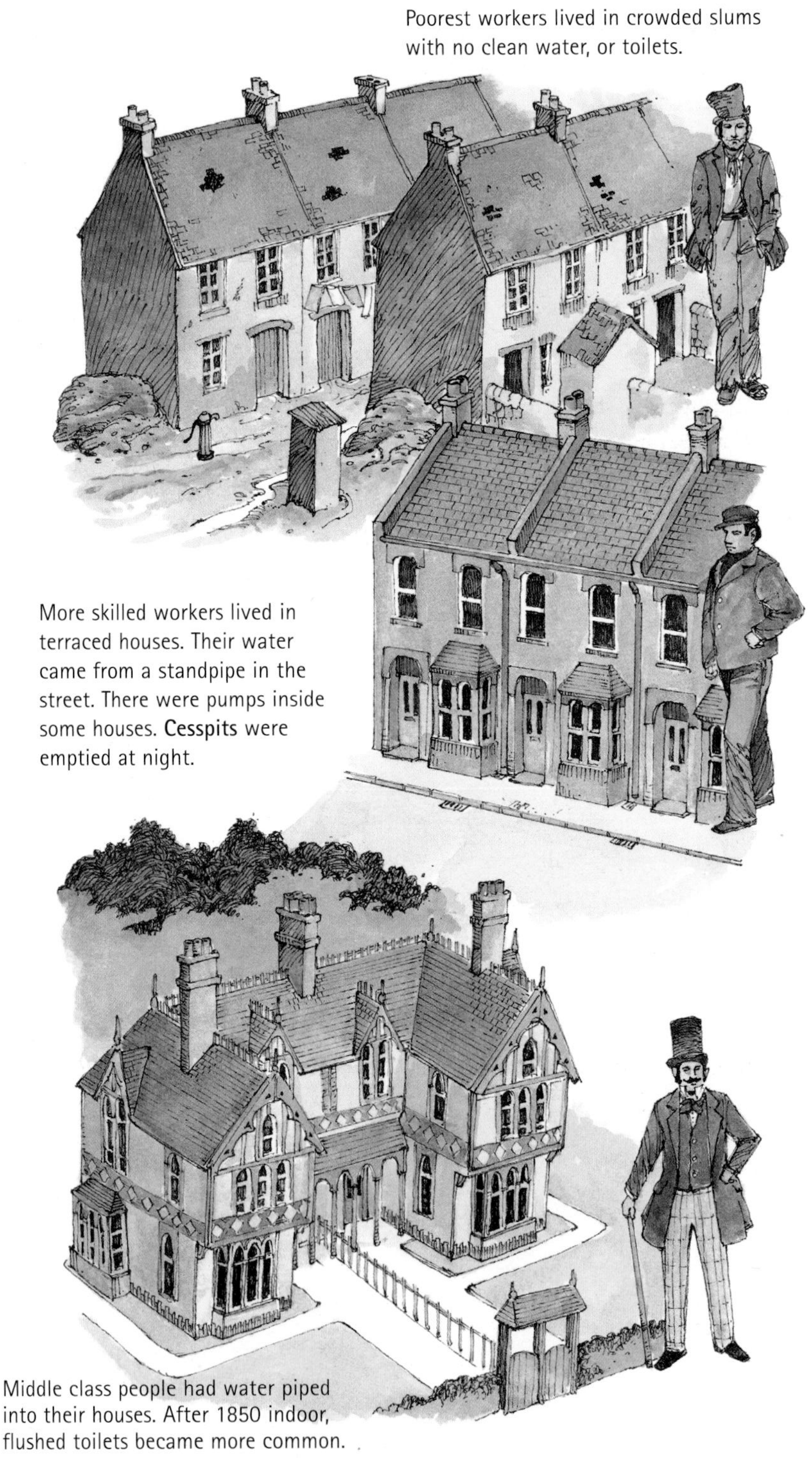

Poorest workers lived in crowded slums with no clean water, or toilets.

More skilled workers lived in terraced houses. Their water came from a standpipe in the street. There were pumps inside some houses. **Cesspits** were emptied at night.

Middle class people had water piped into their houses. After 1850 indoor, flushed toilets became more common.

▲ **SOURCE A** Health by social class.

Average life expectancy was particularly low because deaths amongst children were very high. This is called 'infant mortality' and happens because babies are particularly vulnerable to diseases.

More evidence comes from the terrible epidemics of killer diseases which swept through the crowded slums of these industrial towns and cities.

Why was urban life so unhealthy?

Compared with today people in the eighteenth and nineteenth centuries lived in less healthy conditions. These conditions were worse in the towns than in the countryside (see Source B). The life expectancy of workers in the towns was lower than that of rural workers. Town life had always been unhealthy but it became much more unhealthy during the Industrial Revolution, before it slowly improved after the middle of the nineteenth century. So, improvements are not always continuous, sometimes there is **regression**.

One city - different lives

Remember - people's health varied, depending on social class. By the middle of the 19th century clear social divisions in housing and health could be seen in different parts of an industrial city.

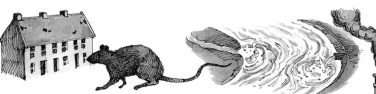

Poorly built houses were damp and infested with disease-carrying animals and insects.

Lack of sewage systems led to pollution of rivers and wells.

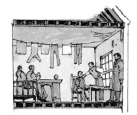

Overcrowded accommodation spread infectious diseases.

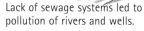

Poor working conditions left people exhausted and less able to recover from illness.

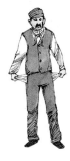

Low wages meant poor people were badly nourished and more likely to catch diseases.

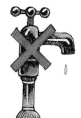

Lack of piped water meant unclean sources had to be used.

▲ **SOURCE B** Factors which made urban life particularly unhealthy.

QUESTION

What posed the greatest threat to the health of people in industrial towns and cities?

KEY WORDS

cesspit – a pit where human waste is dumped

regression – when events do not lead to improvements but get worse

Concluding your enquiry:

Why were British industrial towns so unhealthy? Explain why town life became so unhealthy. Explain why this differed for different classes.

Cholera and its

Epidemics of many diseases killed large numbers of people in the nineteenth century. These included diseases such as typhus, typhoid and cholera. When cholera first reached Western Europe in the nineteenth century, it revealed how little was understood about the causes of infectious diseases.

CHOLERA

Origins: First recorded in India, 400 BC.

Causes: Drinking from water polluted by the excrement or vomit of cholera victims.

Symptoms: Diarrhoea and vomiting. Death is eventually caused by fluid loss.

History: Spread from India along trade routes in 1817 into Southeast Asia, China, Middle East. Spread again in 1824, reached Britain in 1831, America in 1832. Other great outbreaks spreading across the world happened in: 1839, 1865, 1899 and 1961.

There is not the slightest reason for imagining it [cholera] has been **imported** *into the town. It appears to have arisen from disturbances in the* **atmosphere.** *Stopping the trade of the port will encourage the disease by depriving the poor of their bread and placing their families in the depth of misery and distress.*

▲ **SOURCE A** Report by doctors in Sunderland in 1831. They are opposing stopping goods going in and out of the town. This is called a 'quarantine'. Only a few weeks before, the Sunderland Board of Health – set up to prevent disease – had been taken over by local merchants.

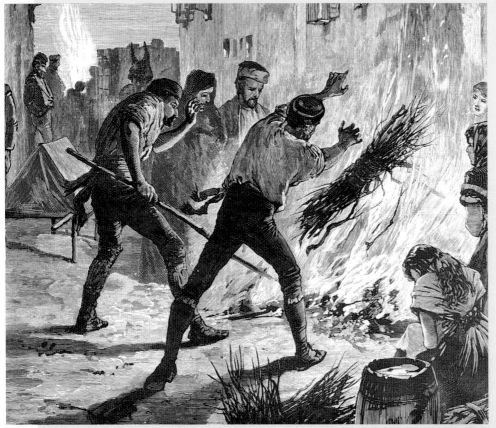

◀ **SOURCE B** Spanish villagers build bonfires in 1865, in order to 'clean the air' to prevent cholera.

causes

Two men attended a cock fight in the afternoon and had supper at a public house with the company who had engaged in this cruel and wicked sport. While at the supper, the townsman was seized with cholera, and was a corpse in about 12 hours. The countryman fell ill as soon as he got home, and within two days was dead. A man from Newcastle, a dreadful swearer and Sabbath breaker, as well as a drunkard, was seized by cholera and died in a few hours.

▲ SOURCE C From the **Methodist** *Magazine*, 1832.

A crowd attacked a surgeon attending a cholera victim. They threw stones and yelled 'medical murderer'. Some maintained that the patient's death was due to the doctor forcing drugs down her throat.

▲ SOURCE D Report of an attack in Edinburgh in 1832.

Some doctors suggested heat. Bleeding was common. One Penzance doctor bled two parients by long cuts in their scalps. Both died.

▲ SOURCE E Reports of treatments carried out in the 1830s.

KEY WORDS

atmosphere –	the air
imported goods –	brought into a country by trade
Methodist –	a Christian group
miasma –	belief in a poisoning of the air thought to cause disease
sabbath breaker –	a person who does not worship God on Sunday

QUESTIONS

1 What does each source suggest was the cause of cholera?

2 Which two sources offer a similar explanation?

3 What reasons might lie behind the point of view in Source A? How does this affect the reliability of this opinion?

4 How might these sources be used as evidence for the continuation of medieval and earlier beliefs in the nineteenth century. Think about:

- beliefs in 'miasma'
- humours
- punishment from God
- blaming unpopular minorities.

☑ EXAM TIP

Question 1 gives practice in comprehension.
Question 2 gives practice in comparing.
Question 3 gives practice in assessing reliability
Question 4 gives practice in using the sources and your own knowledge.

Concluding your enquiry:
Why were British industrial towns so unhealthy?
Which is the better explanation: poor public health, or poor medical knowledge?

enquiry

How scientific was Dr Snow's discovery about cholera?

He marked the locations of the homes of those who had died. From the marks on the map Snow could see that all the deaths had occurred in the Golden Square area. So Snow went down to Broad Street where he suspected one particular pump was the source of the contaminated water. He removed the handle of the pump. The epidemic stopped.

▲ **SOURCE A** R M Henig, *The People's Health*, 1997.

In August 1854 cholera broke out in central London. It is one of the most famous cases of cholera because of the actions of Dr John Snow. Snow believed that cholera was not caused by poisons in the air but by drinking water contaminated by the excrement, or vomit, of a cholera victim. At the time there was great disagreement about the causes of cholera and many experts did not agree with Dr Snow's beliefs.

On Thursday, 7th September, 1854, Dr Snow persuaded the authorities to remove the handle of the water pump on the corner of Broad Street. This was because he believed it was water from this pump that was causing the cholera. Soon after this, the outbreak of cholera stopped.

The triumph of science?

Dr Snow has become famous for carrying out a proper scientific enquiry. There are many accounts of how he:

- mapped where cholera victims lived

- noticed the worst cases were round the Broad Street pump

- removed the handle of the pump to stop the cholera outbreak.

But was it that simple? Was this actually how Dr Snow worked? Did he really stop the 1854 cholera outbreak?

It is supposed that the Broad Street outbreak of cholera was stopped by the closing of the pump. However the outbreak had already reached its climax and had been steadily on the decline for several days before the pump-handle was removed.

▲ **SOURCE B** Rev. Whitehead in 1867. He had carried out his own investigations in 1854. He had discovered that a cesspit was leaking into the Broad Street well. The clothes of a baby who died on 2nd September had been washed and the dirty water poured into the cesspit.

Other observers looked at more detailed maps than Snow's, yet came to different conclusions about the cause of the cholera outbreak. More importantly, Snow came up with his idea before he drew his map. The map did not give him the idea but it confirmed ideas held by several [other] people.

▲ **SOURCE C** *The Lancet* magazine, 2000.

▼ SOURCE D Dr Snow's famous map. He actually drew the map in December 1854, almost three months after the pump handle was removed.

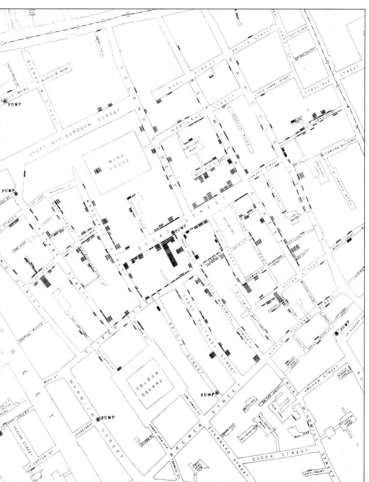

There was nothing in the atmosphere to account for the spread of cholera. He thought he had collected enough evidence to show that in all cases cholera was spread by swallowing some of the excrement of the affected person.

▲ SOURCE E Dr Snow's ideas, reported in *The Lancet* medical magazine, 21st October, 1854.

QUESTIONS

1 Look at Source A and the text. Why is Dr Snow often thought of as being so important? Explain *what* he is said to have done and *why* this was so important.

2 Why might Sources B, C and D make you question this view of him. Think about the methods he actually used and the impact of his actions in 1854.

Concluding your enquiry:
How scientific was Dr Snow's discovery? Explain why Snow's work might not have been as scientific as some have suggested. Explain why he is important anyway.

enquiry

> ## How did industrial towns and cities become safer places in which to live?

What is public health?

One of the great changes that affected health in the nineteenth century was the increase in government responsibility for public health. This is the idea that the government should play a part in preventing diseases.

This is not necessarily the same as the government taking responsibility for curing the sick. Although since the sixteenth century the Poor Law had been used to provide support for very ill people who could not support themselves, this was not the same as providing hospitals and medical treatment for everyone. However, during the nineteenth century, governments stopped believing in the idea of *laissez-faire* with regard to public health. This idea was that governments should *not* intervene in the lives of citizens. Instead, politicians began to get involved in public health. There are two sides to public health:

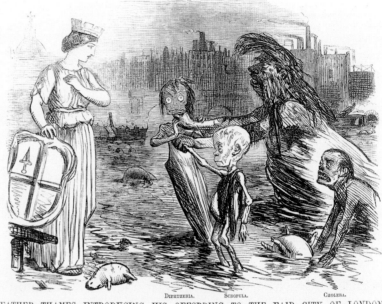

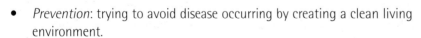
FATHER THAMES INTRODUCING HIS OFFSPRING TO THE FAIR CITY OF LONDON.

▲ **SOURCE A** Cartoon from 1858. It shows that by this time people were beginning to think that the filthy state of cities should be dealt with.

- *Prevention*: trying to avoid disease occurring by creating a clean living environment.
- *Cure*: treating people suffering from particular diseases.

It was prevention that government first became involved with. In fact the possibility of widespread cures for diseases did not even emerge as a possibility until after 1865 when it was first discovered that germs cause illness. Even then it was a long time before governments believed that they were responsible for this aspect of public health.

How did changes in public health begin?

Cholera outbreaks in the 1830s shocked people. Boards of Health were set up in many towns to try to prevent the disease but most were disbanded when the outbreak stopped. Change was slow for many reasons. Before 1835 many towns did not have Town Councils to set up a Board of Health.

> ## ☑ EXAM TIP
>
> The career of Chadwick reminds us that progress in Cure and Prevention does not always advance at the same rate. He is a good example of the role of the individual as a factor for change. Make sure that you understand how in the *short term* Chadwick did not seem successful, but how his work led to *long-term* improvements.

In 1835 the Municipal Corporations Act set up elected town councils who could raise a tax (rates) to pay for street lighting, pavements, fresh water supply and sewage disposal.

In 1838 conditions in London were investigated by Doctors Arnott, Kay and Smith. Their findings were shocking. The Bishop of London argued in the House of Lords that a nationwide survey should be carried out into the health of the poor. It was the start of the 'Sanitary Reform Movement' and the job was given to Edwin Chadwick.

What impact did Edwin Chadwick have on Public Health?

Chadwick believed that Prevention would save money! In 1842 his *Report on the Sanitary Conditions of the Labouring Classes* showed that city-dwellers had a much lower life expectancy than those living in the country. He believed that the cause of this was the filthy living conditions in towns. He did not know exactly how filth caused disease but – like many others – he knew there was some kind of connection.

Chadwick was not interested in curing the sick. He believed towns needed an *arterial water system*. This involved getting clean water into houses, and drains leading from houses into main sewers. These sewers would carry waste away and the liquid manure could be used by farmers rather than dumped in rivers. The sewer pipes should be made of glazed pottery. This would stop leaks and would mean that the pressure of the water would force solid waste along the pipe. He took this idea from a sanitary engineer named John Roe.

Chadwick said that towns should borrow money to pay for this. The rates would then cover this cost over about 30 years.

QUESTIONS

Why was Edwin Chadwick important?

a Describe why public health needed action.

b Describe how government started to take an interest in public health.

c Explain why Chadwick believed public health was important.

d Describe his successes – then his failures.

He believed that one group in each town should look after these changes. He also said cemeteries should be built on the edge of towns and a medical officer should confirm what people died from.

In 1848 a Public Health Act was passed. This set up a national Board of Health for five years and allowed local Boards of Health to be set up. These had power to clean up towns so as to prevent epidemics. However, many towns refused to set up a board, and the Act did not cover London which remained a big problem. The central Board of Health was eventually abolished in 1858. Many powerful groups (such as water companies) opposed Chadwick. Conservative newspapers, like *The Times*, attacked him for trying to force the country to be clean!

How important was Chadwick? He had no interest in curing disease and he would not work with doctors. He wrote in 1842, 'Engineers are needed for the task in hand not the medical profession.' However, he pushed the government into taking action, his new sewage systems improved health and, in some towns the Boards of Health continued their work.

enquiry

Why did governments become involved in public health in the second half of the nineteenth century?

Edwin Chadwick had been attacked because, as *The Times* put it, he was 'bullying' people into being clean. However, during the second half of the nineteenth century governments began to take a greater interest in public health. This changed for a number of reasons:

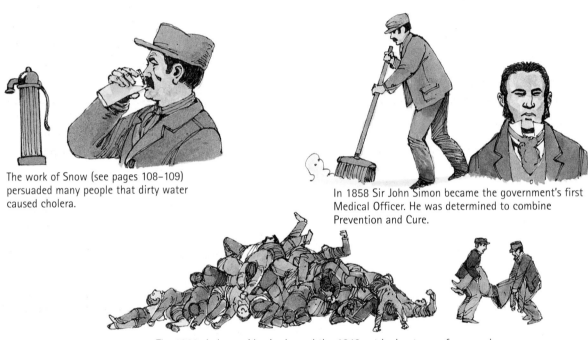

The work of Snow (see pages 108–109) persuaded many people that dirty water caused cholera.

In 1858 Sir John Simon became the government's first Medical Officer. He was determined to combine Prevention and Cure.

The 1866 cholera epidemic showed the 1848 act had not gone far enough. Towns which had ignored it were hit by cholera.

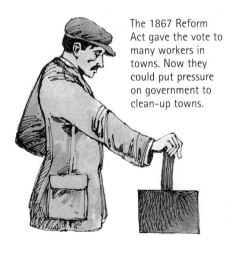

The 1867 Reform Act gave the vote to many workers in towns. Now they could put pressure on government to clean-up towns.

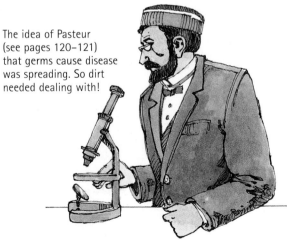

The idea of Pasteur (see pages 120–121) that germs cause disease was spreading. So dirt needed dealing with!

▲ **SOURCE B** The reasons why nineteenth-century governments began to take an interest in public health.

What did the government do?

Between 1866 and 1900 different British governments passed a number of laws to improve public health. Some gave greater power to Local Government to take action. Some made the National Government more involved in public health:

1866 Sanitary Act meant that towns had to appoint inspectors to check water supplies and drainage.

1869 Royal Sanitary Commission recommended that to avoid confusion, all local public health should be the responsibility of one Local Government Board in each area.

1872 Public Health Act split the country into areas inspected by a Medical Officer of Health.

1875 Artisans Dwellings Act gave local authorities power to knock down slums. New Public Health Act cleared up confusion in law.

1884 Royal Commission found most inner city houses were unhealthy.

1890 Housing of the Working Classes Act gave more power to local authorities to clear slums and build new houses.

No less than 29 sanitary measures have been enacted since 1846. These Acts have been made at different times by various people and with different aims.

▲ **SOURCE C** *The Times*, 15th August 1875. This was explaining why the Public Health Act (1875) was so important in making the law more straightforward.

Sir John Simon was more forward thinking than Chadwick, believing that public and private health were complimentary.

▲ **SOURCE D** David Taylor, an historian writing in the book, *Mastering Economic and Social History*, 1988.

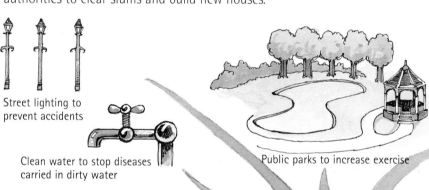

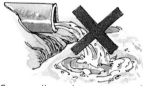

Street lighting to prevent accidents

Clean water to stop diseases carried in dirty water

Public parks to increase exercise

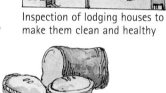

Inspection of lodging houses to make them clean and healthy

Clean food to prevent food poisoning

Responsibilities of local authorities after 1875

Sewage disposal to prevent pollution

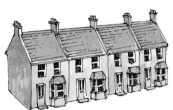

Improving quality of new houses to stop damp and overcrowding

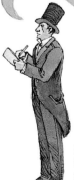

Health and medical inspectors to enforce these rules

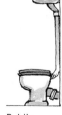

Public toilets to avoid pollution

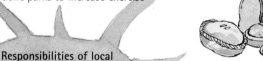

▲ **SOURCE E** The responsibilites of local authorities after 1875.

enquiry

The impact of individual reformers

A number of individuals played a part in persuading the government to improve housing. Queen Victoria's husband, Prince Albert, had 'model houses' built in Hyde Park at his own expense to accompany the Great Exhibition of 1851. He did this to encourage others to take an interest in healthy housing.

George Peabody was an American who provided money to pay for better quality housing for poor people in London.

Octavia Hill worked on projects to build healthier houses for working class people and to provide parks in towns.

The power of philanthropy and the power of parliament

Reformers such as Peabody and Hill are known as 'philanthropists'. This word is used to describe people who love others and who want to do good things to help them.

What these philanthropists did was important because it showed the way forward, it encouraged educated people to take an interest in housing and it encouraged governments to get involved too. The philanthropists encouraged powerful people to think more about their responsibilities to help other people who were less well-off. They also made an impact on poorer people's lives by the changes they made in building healthier housing.

However, there was a limit to what they could achieve as individuals. Their money and resources were limited and they could only help a small number of people. It was only when government became involved after 1860 that great changes started to occur. Governments had the power to change the law, but it was Local Government who had to take on the work of carrying out most of the reforms agreed by parliament in London.

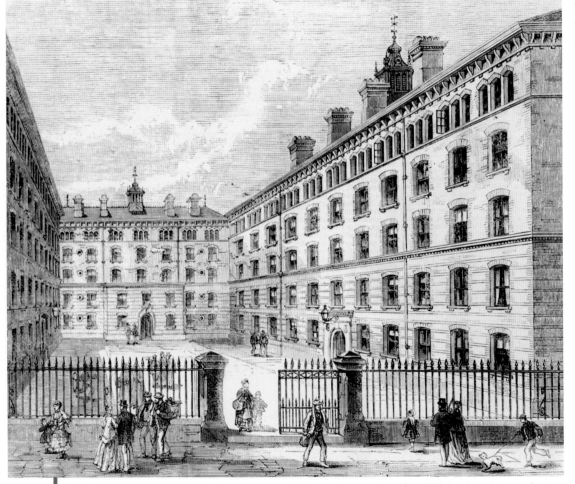

▲ **SOURCE F** Well-built houses in Peabody Square, London. This was one of the projects of the American, George Peabody, who wanted healthier housing for the working class.

Octavia Hill – the impact of an individual reformer

Octavia Hill was born in 1838 in Cambridgeshire. Her father, a banker, was well known for his good work in educational reform. In 1852 Octavia began work in London teaching poor children. In 1864 she persuaded the artist John Ruskin to help her in a scheme to improve the housing of the poor. In 1865 he helped her buy three houses. Her aim was to improve the quality of the houses, make them clean and healthy and to stop overcrowding. She also set up training and education schemes for her tenants. This idea soon spread to other towns in Britain and Ireland and to the USA and European countries.

She worked hard to persuade the government to pass the Artisans Dwellings Act in 1875, which gave power to Local Government to knock down slums. In 1895 she was one of the founders of the National Trust.

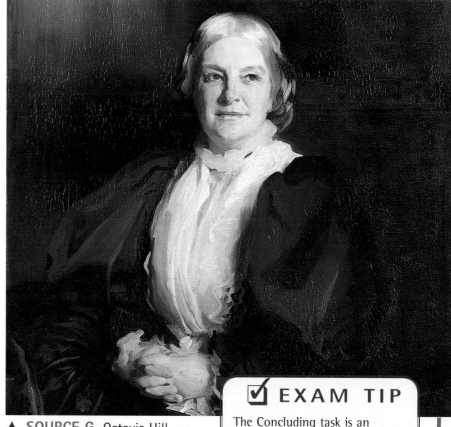

▲ **SOURCE G** Octavia Hill.

QUESTION

Imagine you are a member of the government in 1900. Look back over the nineteenth century, explain why governments in the second half of the nineteenth century became more involved in public health than governments in the first half of the century. In your answer you should:

- explain why governments were at first slow to get involved
- explain reasons why this changed
- decide which reason you think was the most important one
- describe what the government did between 1860 and 1900
- conclude by describing how Public Health improved as a result of what the government did.

☑ **EXAM TIP**

The Concluding task is an example of a Paper 1, Section A question. Say whether you *agree* or *disagree* with the point of view and always back-up your answer with relevant evidence. Do not just give your own point of view without any back-up!

Concluding your enquiry:

How did industrial towns become safer places in which to live?

'Government was more important than individuals in making industrial towns healthier.' Use the information in this Enquiry to say why you *agree*, or *disagree*, with this view.

Public health in

Nineteenth-century towns and cities

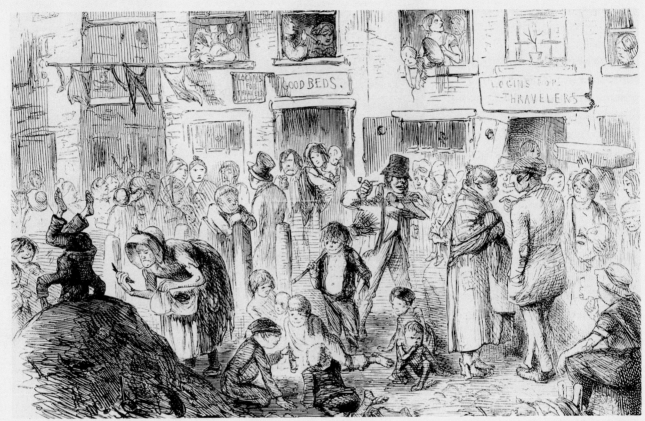

▲ **SOURCE A** *A Court for King Cholera*
This cartoon was published in the magazine *Punch* in September 1852. *Punch* was a magazine that commented upon political and social issues using satire and cartoons. Cholera had struck Britain again in 1848, the same year that the First Public Health Act was passed. Although the Act provided for improved water supplies and sewage disposal it was not compulsory.

Things to notice in the cartoon:

- the pile of sewage in the street
- the woman collecting from the pile
- the crowded street
- the crowded rooms
- children playing with a dead rat
- 'Logins (lodgings) for thravelers (travellers)'
- common lodging houses were overcrowded and very insanitary
- the slum buildings held up by wooden beams between them
- the child's coffin.

☑ **EXAM TIPS**

You will need to use and evaluate sources for Question 1 of Paper 1 in the exam. There will be a variety of sources – pictures, written and statistical. You will need to use both source skills and your own knowledge to reach the highest levels in the marking scheme and, therefore, the highest marks.

Britain

The Board of Health has fallen. We prefer to take our chance of cholera than to be bullied into health. Everywhere the board's inspectors were bullying, insulting and expensive. They entered houses and factories insisting on changes relating to the habits or pride of the masters and occupants. There is nothing a man hates so much as being cleaned against his will, or having his floors swept, his walls whitewashed, his pet dungheaps cleared away, all at the command of a sort of sanitary bumbailiff. Mr Chadwick set to work everywhere and Master John Bull was scrubbed and rubbed till the tears came to his eyes.

◀ **SOURCE B** This was written by the editor of *The Times*, (the most influential newspaper of the time) on the 1st August 1854. On 31st July, parliament had voted to dismiss the General Board of Health and get rid of Chadwick.

QUESTIONS

1 What does Source A tell us about public health in Britain in the middle of the nineteenth century?

2 How useful is Source A for an historian studying public health in Britain in the middle of the nineteenth century?

3 How reliable is Source B for understanding opposition to Edwin Chadwick and his ideas for the reform of public health in Britain in the middle of the nineteenth century.

4 Source A shows that filthy conditions still occurred in British cities after the Public Health Act of 1848.

   Source B says that Britain (Master John Bull) was cleaned as a result of Chadwick's work. Does this mean that the sources contradict each other?

5 Edwin Chadwick's ideas for public health reform were a total failure. How far do you agree with this interpretation? Use the sources and your own knowledge to explain your answer carefully.

KEY WORDS

pet dung heaps –	'favourite' (rather than pet animals)
bumbailiff –	a person who tracked down debtors and sent them to prison
Master John Bull –	Britain

enquiry

Should Edward Jenner be given the credit for defeating smallpox?

Edward Jenner is famous as the man who discovered a way to prevent people catching the dreaded disease smallpox. But is it as simple as that? How much credit should Jenner get for helping rid the world of this disease?

What is smallpox?

Smallpox is an infectious disease. When it is breathed into the lungs it leads to headaches, fever, and an outbreak of sores ('pustules') which can cover the face and body. Of those who got the disease about 25% died from it. Most of the remainder were scarred for life and many went blind. It was a hated and feared disease that for centuries filled people with horror and dread.

The fight against smallpox

By the Middle Ages a way of preventing smallpox, called 'variolation', was used in China and India. This involved introducing pus, or scabs, from a person with smallpox to a healthy person. In China powdered scabs were blown up a person's nose. Giving a person a small dose of a disease to prevent them developing the full form is called 'inoculation'. It causes a person to develop a mild form of the disease but builds up resistance in the body to prevent them catching the full - killer - form of the illness.

News of this method first reached Britain in 1714. One person who made the idea famous was Lady Mary Montague. Her husband was the British ambassador in Turkey where she first came across the method. She had suffered from smallpox as a child and in 1718 had her son inoculated. The idea spread. In 1721, after it had been tried out on volunteer prisoners in Newgate Prison, London, it was used on the wife of the Prince of Wales.

But the method had problems. Some people actually caught smallpox from the inoculation and died. In 1783 the son of King George III died this way. Nevertheless it was less risky than smallpox itself.

> *Future generations will only know by history that smallpox existed and that it was destroyed by you.*

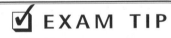 **SOURCE A** US President Thomas Jefferson, speaking about Jenner's work in 1806.

> *Strictly speaking he did not discover vaccination but was the first person to do it scientifically and made it popular. Jenner had been trained in the scientific method and in his studies on vaccination was able to confirm his hypotheses by means of experimentation and observation.*

▲ **SOURCE B** American College of Physicians website, 1997.

☑ EXAM TIP

You can use Jenner, like Snow, as an example of a person who knew *how* his prevention worked, not *why*.

The story of Edward Jenner

Edward Jenner was a Gloucestershire doctor who noticed that milkmaids who caught cowpox (a non-fatal disease) from their cows did not catch smallpox. Jenner was interested in scientific methods and decided to experiment. In 1796 he took pus from a cowpox sore on a girl named Sarah Nelmes and placed it in two small cuts in the arm of an eight-year-old boy named James Phipps. Six weeks later he did the same with smallpox but James showed no reaction. The cowpox had prevented him catching smallpox. Jenner called this vaccination, from the Latin word '*vaca*' (cow).

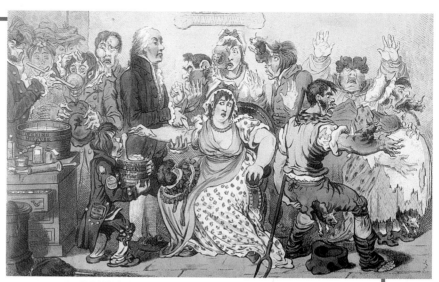

▲ **SOURCE C** A cartoon showing some people's panic about vaccination when it was first introduced.

At first there was lots of criticism of Jenner's idea. Ignorant people thought they would turn into cows! Doctors who were making money from inoculation were angry. Many educated people rejected it because it was different from what people had thought before.

But this changed. By 1800, 100,000 people had been vaccinated worldwide. It was effective without the dangers of inoculation. In 1805 Napoleon of France had his army vaccinated. The use of vaccination continued to spread. In 1980 The World Health Organisation declared that smallpox had finally been removed from the world! It was a triumph for the work started by Jenner.

Should Jenner get the credit for the discovery of vaccination?

In 1765 Dr Fewster of Thornbury in Gloucestershire had written to the Medical Society in London noting that people who had cowpox seemed not to catch smallpox. Thornbury is only a short distance from where Jenner lived at Sodbury.

Then, in 1774, Benjamin Jesty, a farmer from Yetminster in Dorset, vaccinated his wife and sons with pus from a cow with cowpox. He did this because he had seen how two of his servants who had had cowpox nursed two boys with smallpox but did not catch the disease.

So, what was Jenner's contribution?

Jenner had such an impact because he proved his theories through the use of scientific methods and experiments:

- His work on James Phipps was carefully recorded and he published his results.

- In 1799 he carried out a national survey which showed people who had suffered from cowpox did not catch smallpox.

Because of this, the idea spread in a way that it had not done before. Jenner did not invent the idea. But he made other doctors notice it!

QUESTION

Read Source A. What is Jenner given credit for? How does Source B differ? Why?

Concluding your enquiry:
Should Edward Jenner be given the credit for defeating smallpox?
Why was Jenner important?
Why were other people important too?
Decide who was most important.
Show how all were needed to defeat smallpox.

---

enquiry

Why was Pasteur's work a turning point in medicine?

Jenner and Snow did not know *why* diseases spread. All this changed with the work of Louis Pasteur. Pasteur was Professor of Chemistry at the Faculty of Science in Lille, in France. Here he became interested in the problems being experienced by local wine growers. They had difficulties in producing wine of a consistent quality. At times it became sour. Pasteur's use of microscopes led him to discover that specific **micro-organisms** caused wine to go off. If heated these micro-organisms died. This heating became known as 'pasteurising'.

This discovery led him to take an interest in discussions going on between a number of scientists over what caused things to rot and decompose. Many scientists still believed in a Greek and Roman idea called 'spontaneous generation'. According to this idea small organisms suddenly appeared from nowhere. Pasteur was not convinced. His work so far led him to believe that micro-organisms came from other micro-organisms. He conducted a number of scientific experiments:

- He showed that the yeast that caused wine to ferment did not spontaneously appear - but actually came from the skin of the grape. He demonstrated that grape juice taken from under the skin did not ferment.

- He proved that air carried dust and **microbes** which caused contamination. He showed that cleaner air from mountains caused less growth in containers of **fermentable solutions**.

- He used a special shaped swan-necked flask to keep fermentable juice sealed from air and dust. He then allowed air in – but no dust. The juice remained sterile, with no micro-organisms growing in it. It was the dust not the air that caused the growth of micro-organisms.

By 1865 Pasteur was sure diseases were caused by micro-organisms, or germs. His work was to have a great impact on surgery and public health. In England the surgeon Lister was so impressed by Pasteur's idea that he began to clean his bandages and instruments and sprayed antiseptic solutions during his operations to kill germs.

KEY WORDS

fermentable solutions – a mixture on which microbes can feed and grow

microbes – tiny, living creatures, (micro-organisms). Some of which cause disease

There is now no circumstances known in which it can be proved that microscopic beings came into the world without germs.

▲ SOURCE A Pasteur after his experiments with the swan-necked flask.

This water, this sponge, with which you wash or cover a wound may carry germs which have the power of multiplying rapidly in the tissues. I would use only bandages and sponges previously exposed to a temperature of 130° - 150°Celsius.

▲ SOURCE B Pasteur to the Academy of Medicine, Paris, 1878, suggesting how his discovery could change medical practice.

☑ EXAM TIP

After the theory of the Four Humours, the Germ Theory is the next turning point in the history of medicine. Make sure you understand why.

The battle against anthrax, chicken cholera and rabies

The German scientist Robert Koch and the French scientist Casimir Davain had earlier claimed to have discovered the 'bacillus', or germ which caused the disease anthrax. This killed many sheep and cattle a year. Pasteur carried out experiments which confirmed it was this bacillus that caused the disease.

While doing this work on anthrax, chance led to a great discovery. Pasteur had found that chicken cholera bacillus would kill a healthy bird in two days. But one summer containers of this bacillus were left on shelves. Injected into birds, they no longer killed them. However, when the birds were injected with fresh chicken cholera they still did not die. Pasteur realised he had found a new vaccine (see the work of Jenner, on pages 118–119). Soon tests showed that he could follow the same technique and make vaccinations for anthrax and rabies.

Pasteur was reluctant to test his rabies vaccine on people, but in 1886 a young boy, Joseph Meister, was brought to Pasteur having been bitten by a dog with rabies. The boy faced certain death. Pasteur vaccinated him and he survived. By the time Pasteur died, in 1895, he had become an international hero. His Germ Theory had transformed the battle against infectious disease by leading to the development of preventative vaccines.

QUESTIONS

1 Pasteur's discoveries were made through a combination of:

- scientific methods

- scientific equipment

- using ideas of others

- chance.

Explain how each played a part in his discoveries.

2 Using the **key events** in Source C, explain how and why each of Pasteur's discoveries led him onto new discoveries.

▼ **SOURCE C** The key events in Pasteur's discoveries.

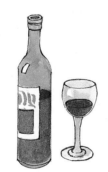

Discovered that microbes caused wine to ferment.

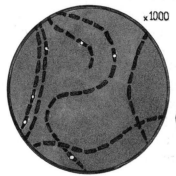

Developed Germ Theory to explain causes of disease.

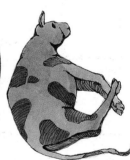

Proved bacillus – found by Koch and Davain – caused anthrax.

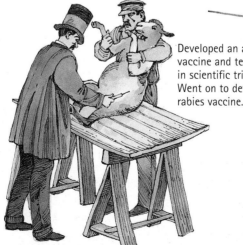

Developed an anthrax vaccine and tested it in scientific trials. Went on to develop a rabies vaccine.

By accident found cholera bacillus could be made into a vaccine.

Concluding your enquiry:

Why was Pasteur's work a turning point? Explain why the Germ Theory was so important.

enquiry

Who should get the credit for discovering the cause of cholera?

Case Study

Robert Koch

Koch is world famous as the German scientist who, in 1882, discovered the *Tubercle Bacillus* which causes tuberculosis and, in 1884, discovered *Vibrio Cholerae*, the germ which causes cholera. Koch was interested in Pasteur's Germ Theory and used it to search for the causes of disease. After the Franco-Prussian War (1870–71) he and Pasteur were rivals just as their different countries were.

In 1883 Koch studied cholera in Egypt. He and his fellow scientists found a comma-shaped microbe in the intestines of cholera victims. In 1884 he continued his work in India, where he was able to prove that this microbe was always found in cholera victims. In 1884 Koch and his team returned to Germany where they were treated as heroes, but it was not easy to persuade other scientists. In 1885 an international conference refused to examine the findings of Koch. Finally his ideas were taken up by other researchers – such as Pasteur in France – and accepted. This was partly because what Koch was claiming fitted in with what Pasteur had earlier discovered. Koch found that certain coloured dyes were attracted to bacteria and stained them. This made it easier to see them. Later, other scientists in the early twentieth century (such as Paul Ehrlich, see page 142) would experiment with dyes which killed the germs. This would lead to ways of not just *preventing* disease but also *curing* it when it affected people. Koch grew germs in agar jelly (made from seaweed, it provided food for microbes) in dishes, devised by Richard Petri, and used special lenses which allowed him to photograph germs through a miscoscope. Using Koch's methods, other researchers identified the causes of tetanus (1884), pneumonia (1886), meningitis (1887), plague (1894) and dysentery (1898). Finally Koch received the Nobel Prize for Medicine in 1905.

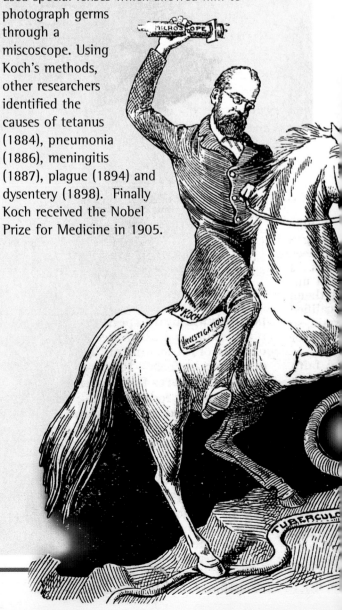

Case Study

Filippo Pacini

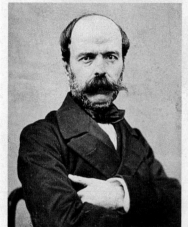

An Italian scientist, Pacini, worked at the Medical School at Pistoia and at the University of Florence. When cholera appeared in Pistoia in 1854 he cut up and examined the internal organs of cholera victims. Through his microscope he found a germ, or 'bacillus', in their intestines which was shaped like a tiny comma. He published his findings in 1854.

His work was completely ignored by the scientific community. In later work he explained – correctly – why cholera caused death and how victims could be treated with injections of sodium chloride in water. We now know this to be a useful treatment to replace liquids lost due to cholera. Pacini accepted the Germ Theory published by Pasteur and insisted that cholera was contagious. His work was still ignored by scientists who believed cholera was caused by miasma. Lack of publicity meant researchers such as Koch did not hear of Pacini's work. However, in 1965 the name of the cholera germ was officially changed to *Vibrio Cholerae Pacini 1854* in honour of the person who first discovered it.

◄ **SOURCE A** Cartoon showing Koch as the winner over infectious diseases.

▼ **SOURCE B** A magnified cholera bacillus.

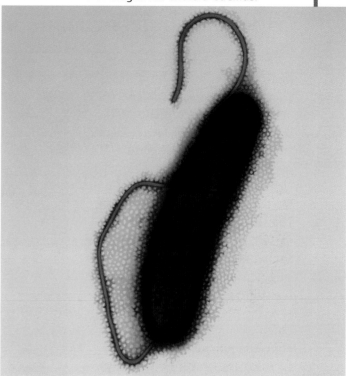

QUESTIONS

1 Who deserves the credit for identifying the cause of cholera: Pacini or Koch?

2 Who deserves the credit for making people *change their minds* about the cause of cholera: Pacini or Koch?

3 What does this tell you about:

  a The way scientific research is not always limited to one person's work.

  b The importance of persuading others to accept new ideas.

  c The difference between 'discovery' and 'acceptance of the discovery'.

Concluding your enquiry:
Who should get the credit for combating cholera? Present the case for Pacini, then for Koch, and decide.

enquiry

How did surgery change in the nineteenth century?

There are two great problems to be overcome in surgery: pain and infection. In the nineteenth century advances in surgery finally overcame these problems.

Surgery involves an entry into the body which causes great pain. The shock of this pain could kill a person, or cause them to writhe in agony, making it impossible for a surgeon to operate successfully. As a result the operation designed to save the person could kill them. Complex operations deep in the body were almost impossible to carry out successfully. The only operations that were carried out with some success were:

- amputations

- trephining

- removing small tumours.

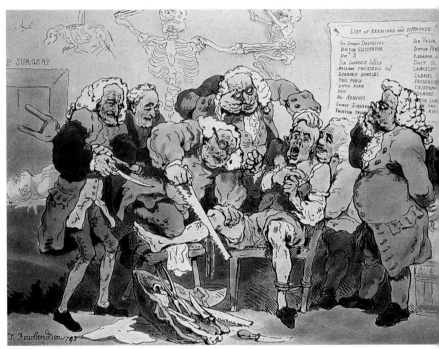

▲ **SOURCE A** An operation in 1793 before anaesthetics.

What was needed, if surgery was to advance, was some way of easing a patient's pain in order to give the surgeon more time to operate. This is known as an anaesthetic. In the 1840s a number of surgeons experimented with different forms of anaesthetics.

The pioneers of anaesthetics

- **Humphry Davy**, in 1799, in England, accidentally discovered that nitrous oxide (laughing gas) eased pain but kept a person conscious.

- **Crawford Long**, in America, noticed that people breathing ether – which was sometimes used for fun at parties in the nineteenth century – did not suffer pain. In 1842 he was the first surgeon to use ether in an operation that took place at Jefferson, Georgia. But he did not publish a report on his discovery until 1849.

- **Horace Wells**, a dentist in the USA, used nitrous oxide in 1844–45 to extract a tooth.

- **William Morton**, another American dentist, experimented with ether in 1846 to remove a tooth. It had a longer lasting effect than nitrous oxide.

- **John Warren**, in 1846, used ether to help remove a growth from a patient's neck in an operation at Massachusetts Hospital, USA.

- **Robert Liston**, another American, used ether in 1846 when amputating a patient's leg.

- **James Simpson**, in Edinburgh, Scotland, used chloroform in 1847 to ease childbirth pain. He preferred it to ether which irritated a patient's lungs and gave off an inflammable gas. He began to use it for general surgery. It soon replaced ether in most European operations.

Opposition to anaesthetics

Some surgeons opposed Simpson's use of chloroform because they were unsure about its effects and how much should be given. Used in the wrong amounts, it could kill. Others believed it was unnatural to stop pain in childbirth. Some thought God meant it to be painful. In spite of this opposition, the case for chloroform slowly advanced and became unstoppable after Queen Victoria used it in childbirth.

The queen had chloroform exhibited to her during her last confinement. It acted admirably. Her Majesty was greatly pleased with the effect and she certainly has had a better recovery. I know this information will please you and I have little doubt that it will lead to a more general use of chloroform in the midwifery practice.

▲ **SOURCE B** From a letter written to James Simpson in 1853 by one of Queen Victoria's doctors. Confinement means childbirth.

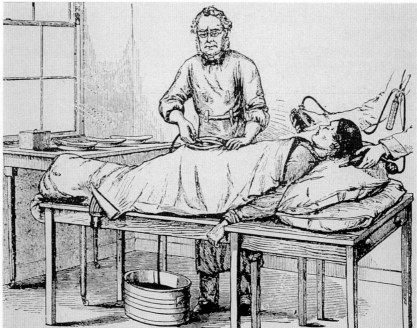

▲ **SOURCE C** An operation after 1847 using chloroform.

QUESTIONS

1   Look at Sources A and C. Describe the two operations. What are the main differences between them?

2   Look at the pioneers of anaesthetics. Who do you think should take the credit for its discovery?

3   Sometimes patients died because surgeons were unsure about the amount of chloroform to use. What other arguments were made against anaesthetics?

4   Read Source B. Why was this a major event in the history of medicine?

5   Explain why anaesthetics are so important and include in your answers:

   • the problems surgeons faced when operatin without them

   • the advantages of using them

   • why loss of blood and infection could still lead to death despite the use of anaesthetics.

☑ **EXAM TIP**

Opposition to anaesthetics was caused by a combination of some religious ideas and some scientific concerns about the dangers of using early anaesthetics when the safe dosage had not been established.

enquiry

'Hospitals should do the sick no harm'!

In today's health service doctors and nurses realise how important it is to avoid passing infections from patient to patient. They try to follow Florence Nightingale's principle that 'Hospitals should do the sick no harm'! Even so, a research study in 1997 estimated that 5,000 people die every year directly from infections caught *in* hospitals and these 'hospital acquired infections' (HAIs) *help cause* the deaths of a further 15,000 people! The greatest cause of 'HAIs' is inadequate hand washing!

Victims of progress?

In the middle of the nineteenth century the need for clean hospital suroundings had not yet been clearly understood because the Germ Theory had not yet been discovered, or accepted. As a result of this, many patients died from infections they picked up in hospitals. This was the dreaded 'hospital sickness' and it was most common in surgical cases. This was because cutting into a person's body allowed infections deep into the body tissues which caused the deaths of many patients.

The problem was actually made worse by the discovery of anaesthetics. Their use, from about 1846, encouraged surgeons to carry out operations that previously they would not have dared to do! But they carried them out in unhygienic conditions. Dirty clothes – worn during numerous operations – and surgical instruments which had not been sterilised, led to many patients dying from hospital acquired infections. Some surgeons even thought that the dried blood on their aprons was a good thing as it demonstrated how experienced they were in surgery!

The appliance of science

In Scotland the Professor of Surgery in Glasgow, Joseph Lister, had read about Pasteur's Germ Theory. He realised that the infections killing his patients were probably caused by germs. In 1867 he decided to apply the new theory to his own work in the operating theatre. To try to kill these germs he:

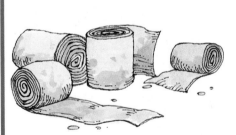

Soaked bandages in carbolic acid.

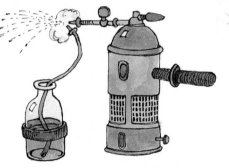

Used a spray that covered the surgeon's hands and the patient with weak carbolic acid.

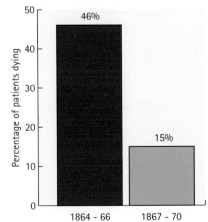

Cleaned the instruments with carbolic acid.

Carbolic acid is an antiseptic and was used to treat sewage as it seemed to reduce the smell. Lister felt it might also be destroying the microbes which caused decay and so thought it might kill germs in the operating theatre. He found it did kill the germs, although the acid spray also damaged the surgeon's hands. Lister's own records showed that the number of deaths following his operations dropped dramatically:

▶ **SOURCE A** Graph showing the percentage of Lister's patients that died after operations before using carbolic acid (1864–66) and when using carbolic acid (1867–70).

Percentage of patients dying

46% (1864 - 66)

15% (1867 - 70)

Same idea – different approach

Carbolic acid created antiseptic conditions because it killed germs, but it was unpleasant to work with and damaged the hands and lungs of surgeons and nurses. In Germany a different but related approach developed. This focused not on killing germs but on keeping them away. This became known as 'aseptic' surgery. The same approach was developed by the US surgeon William S. Halsted, in 1889, after his nurse complained that carbolic acid was ruining her hands. Aseptic surgery led to procedures such as:

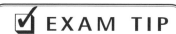

EXAM TIP

The relationship between anaesthetics and antiseptics shows that new discoveries do not always lead to immediate progress and can sometimes cause more problems.

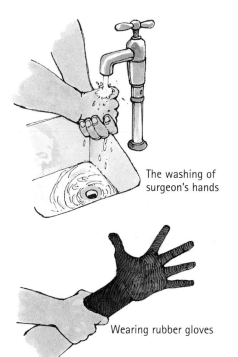

The washing of surgeon's hands

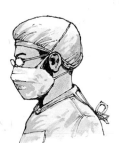

Wearing caps, masks and gowns

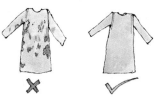

Sterlising surgeons' clothes

Wearing rubber gloves

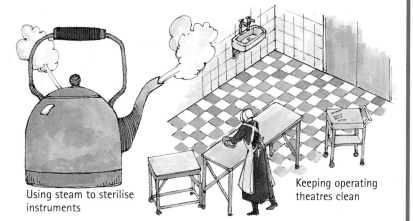

Using steam to sterilise instruments

Keeping operating theatres clean

Despite this progress, preventing blood loss in surgery would remain a problem into the twentieth century.

QUESTION

'Some medical discoveries can lead to progress, while others can lead to problems!' Explain how this was true:

- Think of the impact of the work of Simpson.

- Think of the impact of the work of Lister.

- Explain how each had a different impact on the development of antiseptic surgery.

Concluding your enquiry:

How did surgery change in the nineteenth century?

- describe how anaesthetics changed surgery

- describe how antiseptics changed surgery

- decide which change was most important in helping patients survive surgery and explain why.

Not all science

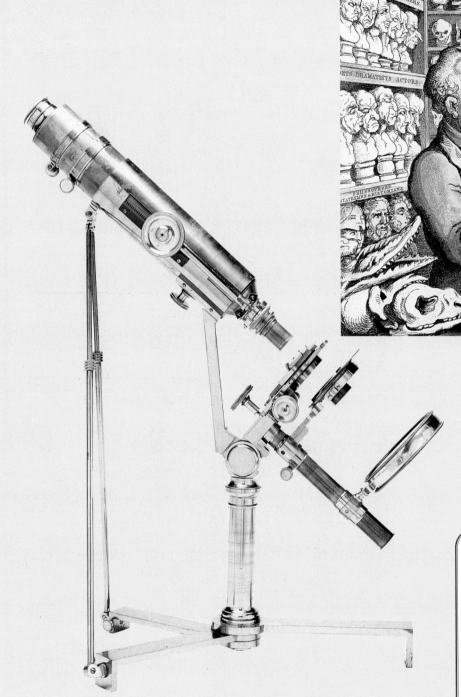

▲ **SOURCE A** F J Gall discussing his theory of phrenology. This was the idea that a person's character could be 'read' from the shape of their head and bumps on their skull.

▲ **SOURCE B** A microscope produced in 1826. It meant very small objects could be seen very clearly.

☑ EXAM TIPS

If an exam question, such as Question 5 on scientific methods, asks you to use sources *and* your own knowledge, first get as much relevant information as you can from the sources, then go on to say what else you know about the issue you are writing about.

led to progress

▶ **SOURCE C** Electricity was used to try to cure tuberculosis in the late nineteenth century.
Such treatment had no effect but was popular anyway.

Any doctor or student coming from the postmortem room must, before entering the maternity wards, wash his hands thoroughly in the basin of chlorinated water placed at the entrance.

▲ **SOURCE D** Notice placed in the Vienna General Hospital by Dr Ignaz Semmelweiss, in 1847.

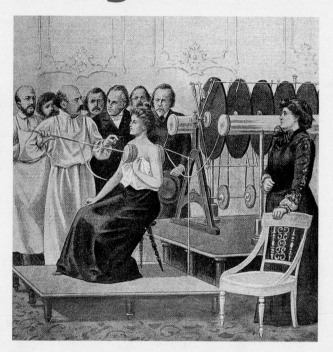

QUESTIONS

1   Why were objects like the microscope in Source B important in changing medical understanding of causes of disease in the nineteenth century?

2   How could Source C be used to show that new technology does not always lead to improvements in medical treatment?

3   Sources A and B are both based on the idea of observation. But can phrenology (SourceA) really provide accurate information about a person's character? Does the microscope in Source B actually identify causes of disease? What can this tell you about the danger of assuming that scientific methods always lead to progress in medicine?

4   Look at Source D. **From your own knowledge** what scientific discoveries were necessary before most doctors were willing to accept Dr Semmelweiss' idea about preventing infection?

5   Read the following interpretation:

'It was scientific methods of careful observation and use of new technology which transformed the treatment of diseases in the nineteenth century.'

Use **the sources in this chapter and your own knowledge** to explain whether you agree or disagree with this view.

KEY WORD

postmortem – means after death. The post mortem room is where bodies are examined to try to discover the cause of death

enquiry

Was it Florence Nightingale who made women important again in medicine?

Florence Nightingale (1820–1910) was a very important person in the development of nursing and medical care. She revolutionised nursing in the second half of the nineteenth century and the changes she made have been at the heart of medical care ever since.

In order to answer our core question we have to understand some important issues:

- How important were women during the period of industrialisation?

- What was Florence Nightingale's contribution and what was its effect on medicine and the role of women in medicine?

- What other changes were there in the role of women in medicine by 1900?

How important were women during the period of industrialisation? The role of women changed during the nineteenth century. Amongst the poor and working class, women maintained their role in medicine. Wives, mothers, sisters and grandmothers acted as nurses, midwives and general carers for family and neighbours in need. 'Wise women' continued to give herbal remedies and charms to cure the illnesses of the poor.

The situation among the rich and at the professional levels of medicine was very different. By 1800 women had largely been excluded from professional medicine in Britain. Until about 1700, upper class women still carried out traditional treatments and saw it as their duty to care for the sick. Scientific medicine had not yet developed enough to provide better cures. There were not yet enough trained doctors to dominate medical care. In the eighteenth century, however, the middle and upper classes turned to physicians for treatment rather than traditional remedies. Since women were denied access to higher education they could not go to universities and so they could not train to be doctors. The universities were exclusively male so men dominated medical training. It became fashionable among the growing middle classes to consult a physician and so the number of trained male doctors increased.

This situation continued well into the nineteenth century when, after much opposition from the medical establishment and a long and bitter struggle, the law allowed women to enter university and be registered as doctors.

QUESTIONS

1 What roles did women play within medicine before the work of Florence Nightingale? In your answer look at the roles played by:

- poor women
- wealthy women.

2 Why was it difficult for some women to challenge the limitations placed on their role in the treatment of the sick?

3 Explain how warfare provided Florence Nightingale with an opportunity to challenge the accepted female role in caring for the sick.

Concluding your enquiry:
In what ways does the life of Florence Nightingale illustrate:

- the difficulties women faced in developing a respectable career in caring for the sick.

- the way in which an individual can change health care.

Biography

FLORENCE NIGHTINGALE

Florence Nightingale was born in Florence, Italy in 1820. At the age of 17 she felt that she was called by God to help other people. After many rows with her family she was allowed, in 1851, to visit Kaiserwerth in Germany where respectable Christian women nursed the sick. In 1853 she was appointed in charge of a private London hospital. When the Crimean war broke out in 1854 she went to Turkey to lead a party of nurses who were to care for sick and wounded soldiers. When the war was over Florence returned to England to work on the reform of the health and medical organisation of the British army. In 1859 she published *Notes on Nursing* and the next year the Nightingale Training School for Nurses opened at St Thomas' Hospital, London. For the next 30 years she worked tirelessly for nurses' training, reform in workhouses and in India. By 1896 she was very ill and confined to bed. Her eyesight failed totally in 1901. She was awarded the Order of Merit by King Edward VII in 1907, the first woman to be so rewarded. She died in her sleep in 1910. Florence Nightingale was admired by many of her contemporaries.

Nobody who has not worked with her daily could know her. They could not have an idea of her strength and clearness of mind, her extraordinary powers joined with her kindness. She is one of the most gifted people that God ever made.

▲ SOURCE A Written in 1857 by Dr John Sutherland, a member of the Royal Sanitary Commission on the Health of the Army. Florence worked on this Commission and proved that many soldiers were dying because of neglect, poor food and disease. She wanted to prevent, as she said, 'Our soldiers enlisting to death in the barracks' by improving conditions. Many politicians and army medical men opposed what they considered to be a revolutionary and cranky idea.

enquiry

How did the role of women in medicine change by 1900?

We see in the medical education of women a horrible attempt to de-sex themselves; in aquiring anatomical knowledge an unhealthy interest in sexual matters and a thirst after forbidden knowledge. In carrying out medical duties they are taking on roles which Nature intended entirely for men.

▲ **SOURCE A** Comments by a male English doctor in the 1850s.

Changing nursing

In 1860 Florence Nightingale set up the first training school for nurses. Her idea spread and further training schools were established. In addition, as new hospitals were being designed, people were beginning to follow her advice on the best way to build wards. However, there was some resistance to new ideas in nursing. In 1879 there was a huge dispute at Guy's Hospital in London, when the new **matron**, Miss Burt, insisted that nurses and **sisters** should not spend all their time on one ward, but should gain experience on a number of wards. Inspired by Florence Nightingale, Miss Burt hoped to create nurses with a wide range of skills that they could take to other wards and hospitals. In 1879 a letter signed by all the doctors and nurses in the hospital protested against her ideas! Eventually they were introduced but only after a struggle.

Women doctors

Elizabeth Blackwell was born in Bristol but had to go to Geneva College, New York, in order to train as a doctor. She qualified in 1847, and in 1857 opened the New York Infirmary for Poor Women and Children, staffed entirely by women. In 1869 she returned to London to start a school of medicine for women. Before this, news of her achievement encouraged a British woman, Elizabeth Garrett-Anderson, to do the same. During the 1860s she worked as a nurse and attended lectures at the Middlesex Hospital. From 1861–65 she applied to every medical school to train as a doctor but she was refused. Eventually she trained privately and passed the exams to become a doctor but faced huge opposition. Male students had protested at her attending lectures. The Colleges of Surgeons and Physicans (the groups which controlled entry to these jobs) refused to accept her. Only after a court case was she able to practise medicine. In 1865 she was accepted as a doctor by the Society of Apothecaries and soon had a large practice in London.

Other women faced the same opposition. Six, led by Sophia Jex-Blake, completed their medical studies at the University of Edinburgh but the university refused to give them their degrees! They had to complete their studies in Dublin, or in Switzerland. Sophia founded the London School of Medicine for Women in 1874.

It was not until 1876 that a change in the law opened up all medical qualifications to women.

She is endeavouring to centralise all nursing arrangements in her office and is destroying the position and authority of the old and trusted ward sisters.

▲ **SOURCE B** From a letter written by a nurse about Miss Burt, to the authorities running Guy's Hospital, London, in 1880.

☑ **EXAM TIPS**

As well as describing general changes the examiners will expect you to know about the influence of individuals too. Make sure you understand why Nightingale, Blackwell and Garrett-Anderson were important in changing the role of women in medicine.

Why did some men oppose women doctors?

They claimed:

- Women were too emotional.

- Women were not intelligent enough.

- Women should not do traditional men's jobs.

- Women should not have authority over men.

- Women could not cope with the hard work and responsibility.

The position in 1900

By 1900 the nursing profession had changed greatly as a result of the ideas of the nineteenth century. It was a respectable occupation for women, with high standards and clear aims. The care of the sick had improved greatly. In 1901 there were 68,000 trained nurses in Britain, whereas in 1850 there had been none. On the other hand nurses were very much under the control of doctors who were mostly male. It would be many years into the twentieth century before a significant number of women trained as doctors. Nevertheless there was now no legal reason why they could not do so. This meant that it was only a matter of time before further changes took place.

▼ **SOURCE C** Nurses before and after Florence Nightingale.

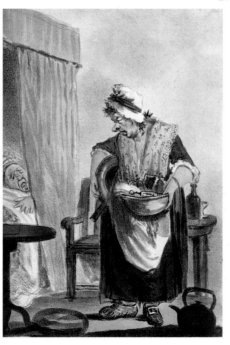
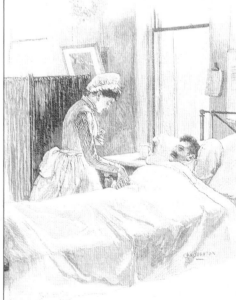

QUESTIONS

1 Read Source A and the text. Explain why many men were opposed to women becoming doctors.

2 Read Source B and the text. Why did some nurses oppose the spread of new ideas about nursing?

3 Do you think the person who drew Source C was for or against the new ideas in nursing? Explain your answer.

Concluding your enquiry:
How did the role of women in medicine change? Describe changes in nursing and in medical training. Explain why there was opposition to these changes. Decide how much had changed by 1900.

review

What progress was made in the industrial world 1700–1900?

To make sense of the extent of changes in the late eighteenth and nineteenth centuries we need to recognise that it was not spread evenly across health and medicine. By far the greatest strides were made in *prevention* of disease. Progress in the *cure of disease* was not so great.

Most of these changes were made possible by a new understanding of life and how to study and explain events. This scientific way of putting forward ideas and testing them by experiments led to great advances in understanding the causes of disease and its treatment.

Prevention and Cure

Prevention

- The development of public health responsibilities by governments had a huge impact on disease and its prevention.

- Scientific discoveries such as vaccination and the Germ Theory led to progress in preventing the spread of disease. These finally ended beliefs in spontaneous generation of germs and in humours causing illness which had been accepted in 1800.

- Improvements in the administration of nursing and in hospitals reduced the spread of disease amongst the sick.

Cure

- Progress began to be made in identifying dyes which, as well as being attracted to and staining disease-causing microbes, could also kill them.

☑ EXAM TIP

Make sure you understand that, for all the progress achieved by 1900, the greatest changes were in the prevention of disease. The greatest changes in the cure of disease did not take place until the twentieth century.

Causes of change

Look at the following areas which led to changes in health and medicine in the late eighteenth and nineteenth centuries. They remind you that a number of different factors combined to lead to changes.

Under each 'area' some of the key people and events have been listed. For each, look back through this book and your work and say how they, or it, changed health/medicine. Identify whether the change affected prevention of disease, or cure of disease. If you can think of any other individuals, or events, add them to the list.

Role of Education, Science and Technology
- Scientific methods of enquiry
- New equipment (e.g. microscopes)

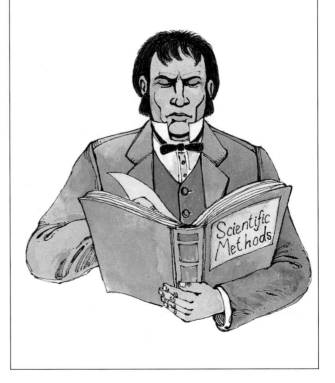

Role of Individuals

- Jenner and vaccination
- Chadwick and public health
- Simpson and anaesthetics
- Snow and cholera
- Nightingale and nursing
- Garrett-Anderson and women doctors
- Hill, Peabody and housing
- Lister and antiseptics
- Pasteur and the Germ Theory
- Koch and identifying disease-causing microbes

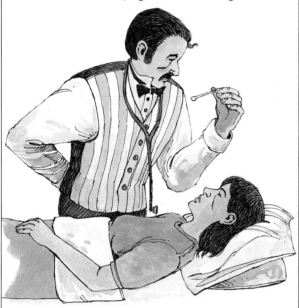

Role of Government

- Conditions in towns and cholera epidemics
- public health
- Crimean War

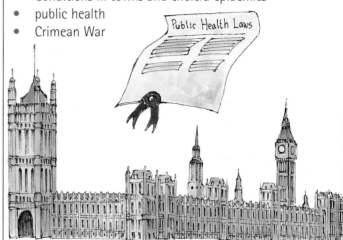

Role of Religion

- Christian reformers founding new hospitals
- Opposition to anaesthetics
- Committed Christian, Florence Nightingale, cared for the sick

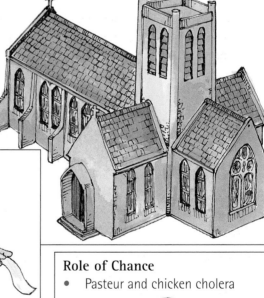

Role of Warfare

- The Crimean War

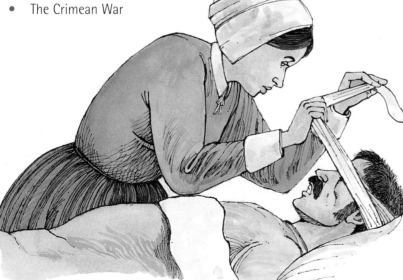

Role of Chance

- Pasteur and chicken cholera

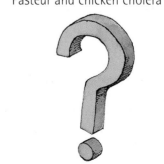

overview

Welcome to the Modern World

What special problems face historians who study the modern world?

In the next 50 years there will be many changes to the world in which you live. In studying the modern world historians face problems. They are studying events of the time in which they live. People alive today have first-hand memories of these events and will want to preserve what they remember. Being so close to events makes it difficult to decide which are the most important. You might think that only time will tell but a good historian will examine the evidence carefully and consider it in the light of events from earlier centuries before making a judgement about what is and what is not important. A twentieth-century historian commented that 'history is the relationship between the past, the present and the future'. The future has not happened yet and the present is gone in a split second so we can only study the past to understand the other two.

What are the key features of medicine in the modern world?

One of the biggest forces for change in the modern world is technology. This allows huge amounts of information to be processed, and sent anywhere within minutes. In 1900 the motorcar, aeroplane and telephone had just been invented and very few people owned them. By 2000 everyone, even in the poorest areas of the world, was affected by this information and communication revolution. Food and medicine could be sent anywhere to combat famine and disease. Sick people could be transported to hospitals in other countries for treatments not available in their own. Doctors and scientists from all over the world could exchange ideas using the Internet. Technology could also pollute and destroy the world like never before.

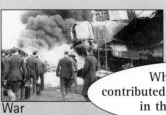
War

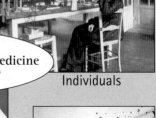
Individuals

What factors have contributed to changes in medicine in the modern world?

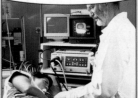
Chance

Science and Technology

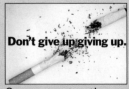

Don't give up giving up.

Government action

Study the examples below and think about the factor which caused each discovery:

Canal fever

In 1904 the French had to give up trying to build the Panama Canal because over 20,000 workers had lost their lives to yellow fever. They turned the project over to the USA. An army doctor, William Crawford Gorgas, discovered that mosquitoes passed on the disease. He was able to wipe it out within a year and the canal was finished.

Submarines and babies

By 1918 French scientists had developed the sonar (sound navigation and ranging) system. This was installed in submarines and ships to detect other vessels. In the 1950s an English scientist, Ian Donald, discovered he was able to study the shape of an unborn baby's body and internal organs by using this system on the mother's abdomen. We call it ultrasound scanning. It is used to check the health of unborn babies.

Science and surgery

Three American physicists invented and built the first laser in 1960. Arthur Schawlow, one of the inventors, recalled, 'We thought it might have had

▼ SOURCE A An ultrasound scan.

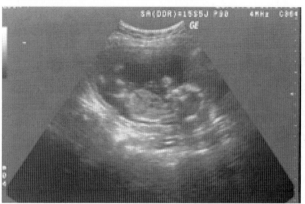

some communications and scientific uses but we had no application in mind. If we had, it might have hampered us and not worked out as well.' Today lasers are widely used in surgery to cut through flesh, to treat many eye problems and to seal off tiny blood vessels to prevent bleeding.

Movies and medicine

In 1978 cities in the USA reported a 60% drop in the number of organs donated for transplant operations. Dr James Cerilli concluded that the motion picture *Coma*, which was about hospital patients murdered so that their organs could be sold for transplants, was at least partly responsible for the drop in organ donations.

☑ EXAM TIPS

Question 2 is a useful revision aid. Examination questions often ask about the factors which brought about or slowed down changes in medicine. Go back through the previous enquiries in the book and make a list of these so that you can use them later on for revision.

QUESTIONS

1   Look at the examples described on this page. Now look at the diagram showing the factors that have contributed to changes to medicine in the modern world.
    For each example note down the factor which helped to make that change in medicine happen.

2   Have any of the factors you have noted down in question 1 helped to bring about changes in medicine at other times in history?

enquiry

Why did governments take action to improve public health in Britain early in the twentieth century?

During the nineteenth century, governments had begun to take an active role in improving the nation's health (see pages 112–117). Government action continued into the new century. It was based on research into the health and living conditions of the poor that shocked many people at the time. Britain had been the most powerful country in the world during the reign of Queen Victoria (1837–1901) but, in 1900, it was facing strong competition from countries such as Germany, France and the USA. As Britain entered the twentieth century the experience of the Boer War taught the government a valuable lesson.

Recruitment for the Boer War (1899–1901) showed that two out of every five of the British men who volunteered to fight were medically unfit. In 1914 recruits in the First World War (1914–18) were found to be similarly unhealthy.

At the same time working men, who had only just gained the right to vote, began trying to influence government to improve their lives. They joined trade unions to gain higher wages and better conditions of work. In 1900 a small group formed their own Labour Party, which hoped to influence the Conservatives and Liberals so that they would use government power to improve the lives of working people and the poor.

How did the work of individuals change government opinions about poverty and health?

Charles Booth *(1840–1916)*

Charles Booth was born in Liverpool on 30th March 1840. Booth's father was head of the Lamport & Holt Steamship Company. When Booth was 22 his father died and he took over the running of the company. He was a good leader and a successful businessman. In 1885 he became angry about a claim made that 25% of the people of London lived in real poverty. Bored with running his successful business, Booth decided to investigate pauperism in the East End of the city. The result of Booth's investigations, *Life and Labour of the People of London*, was published in 1889. Booth's book revealed that the situation in London was even worse than had been claimed. His research suggested that 35% rather than 25% were living in real poverty.

Booth now decided to expand his research to cover the rest of London. He continued to run his business during the day and left his writing to evenings and weekends. In an effort to obtain a comprehensive and reliable survey Booth and his small team of researchers made at least two visits to every street in the city.

Over a 12-year period (1891–1903) Booth published 17 volumes of *Life and Labour of the People of London*. In these books Booth argued that the government should take responsibility for people living in poverty. One of the proposals he made was for the introduction of old age pensions. Booth believed that if the government failed to take action, Britain was in danger of experiencing a socialist revolution.

Whereas many of his researchers, including Beatrice Potter, became socialists as a result of what they discovered while investigating poverty, Booth became more conservative in his views. He was strongly against trade unions and unhappy with the sympathetic treatment unions had received from the Liberal government that took power after the 1906 General Election. Booth gave up his early support for the Liberal Party and joined the Conservative Party. He died in 1916.

David Lloyd George
(1863–1945)

---

and Seebohm Rowntree
(1871–1954)

David Lloyd George was the son of a primary school headmaster in Manchester. When he was only 18 months old his father died so his mother took him to live in Wales with his uncle, who was a local shoemaker and Baptist minister. It was his uncle who made it possible for David to become a solicitor in 1884. He later joined the Liberal Party and was elected as MP for the Welsh town of Caernarvon in 1890. In 1895 he was well known for speaking out against the Conservative government, and at a meeting in Birmingham he was nearly lynched by a crowd because he spoke against the Boer War in South Africa.

Seebohm Rowntree was another successful businessman who took an interest in people who were much poorer than he was. In 1897 he took over his father's successful chocolate-making business in York. His father had been interested in the problem of poverty in Britain and Seebohm decided to carry on his father's work. He spent two years (1899–1901) collecting facts about living conditions in the city of York. In 1901 he published the results in *Poverty: A Study of Town Life*. His main conclusion is shown in Source A on page 140.

Rowntree was a member of the Liberal Party. In 1907 he met and became friends with David Lloyd George. In 1908, with the Liberal Party back in power, Lloyd George became the Chancellor of the Exchequer. He introduced the first British old age pensions and national health insurance. In 1916, during the First World War, he became the Prime Minister but the Liberal Party split over how to run the country during the war and his party was never to govern again during the twentieth century.

Seebohm Rowntree, however, went on to produce many more studies on the lives of working people. He believed that healthy and well-fed workers were also efficient workers. One change that he made in his own company was to increase the pay of his 4,000 workers.

In the 1930s Rowntree carried out a second survey of York, *Progress and Poverty* (1941). He argued that the city had experienced a 50% reduction in poverty since 1901. In 1899 the main cause of poverty had been low wages but in the 1930s it was unemployment. A person at the time said Rowntree's work made him the 'Einstein of the Welfare State'.

Concluding your enquiry:

Why did governments take action to improve public health in Britain early in the twentieth century?

The information in this enquiry suggests that individuals were very important in encouraging government action on poverty and health at the beginning of the century.

Use the information to make a diagram summarising what each individual did and how their actions were connected. What other factors encouraged government action on public health at this time?

Government action and its effects on

In this land of great wealth, during a time of growing prosperity, probably more than a quarter of the population are living in poverty.

▲ **SOURCE A** B S Rowntree, *Poverty: A Study of Town Life*, 1901

We have already reduced personal responsibility by taking away from parents the duty of educating their children. This is now used as an argument for taking away from them the duty of feeding their children. From that it is an easy step to paying for their proper housing. The proposed measure (free school meals for the poorest children) would go far to drain the remaining independence of the parents.

▲ **SOURCE B** *The Times*, 2 January 1905. Not everyone felt that the government should spend taxpayer's money on improving the health and welfare of the poor.

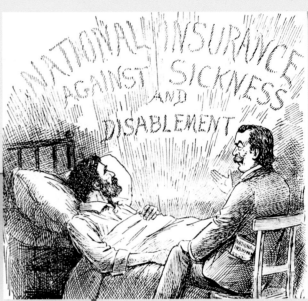

▲ **SOURCE C** A poster produced by the Liberal government seeking support for their policy of compulsory National Insurance in 1911. It shows David Lloyd George explaining his National Insurance Act to a man who is sick in bed. All wage-earners between 16 and 70 would have to join the scheme if they earned less than £160 per year. They would have to pay 4d(2p) per week. The employer would add another 3d(1.5p)and the state 2d(1p). In return the insured worker would receive free medical attention with medicine when they needed it but not hospital treatment. If they could not work they would receive 50p per week for up to 26 weeks.

1906 Education (Provision of Meals) Act
Local Authorities given the power to provide school meals for the poorest children
1908 Old Age Pensions Act
50 pence per week was given to all people over the age of 70
1911 National Health Insurance Act
A compulsory insurance scheme for all workers earning less than £160 per year. When they were sick it allowed them to draw benefit.
1919 Housing Act
Gave local authorities finance so that they could provide 'Homes fit for heroes' after the First World War.
1930 Housing Act
Slums were cleared from many large towns and cities. Local authorities were forced to provide 'council' housing for families whose houses were pulled down.

▲ **SOURCE D** List of Parliamentary acts showing some of the actions taken, by different governments, to improve the health and welfare of poor people in Britain in the early part of the twentieth century.

☑ **EXAM TIP**

When asked 'Do you agree?' in a question always try to give arguments for both sides then come to a conclusion based on the evidence in the sources and your knowledge.

health in early twentieth century Britain

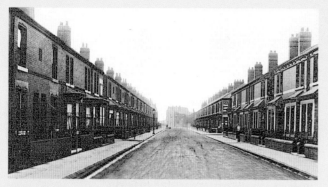

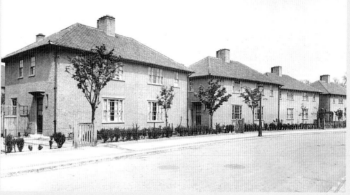

◄ **SOURCE E** A street of terraced houses in Doncaster, South Yorkshire, photographed in 1910. The houses are typical of those built for railway workers in the late nineteenth century. They have two rooms upstairs and two rooms downstairs. There is an outside toilet in a small yard at the back of each house but there is no bathroom.

▲ **SOURCE F** A photograph of an early council estate street in Essex built in the 1920s. Each house would have its own bathroom and inside toilet with gardens at the back and front.

QUESTIONS

1   What can you learn from Source A about the success of government action in the late nineteenth century in improving the health and welfare of people in Britain by 1901?

Explain your answer using Source A, the information on Rowntree and Booth on pages 138–139 and the earlier enquiries on government action in the late nineteenth century.

2   Read Source B and study Source C:

   a Why did some people in the early twentieth century oppose social reforms?

   b How did public health benefit from the Liberal reform shown in Source C?

3   Study Sources E and F. How good are these sources as evidence of the improvement in living conditions for working people in Britain between 1910 and 1930?

4   The 1936 report *Food, Health and Income* referred to in Source G showed that government action in the early twentieth century had failed to improve the health of people in Britain. Do you agree? Use these sources and your knowledge to help you to explain your answer.

Dr John Boyd-Orr was appointed as Director of the Nutrition Institute in Aberdeen, in 1914, at the age of 34. During World War One he served in the Royal Army Corps earning two medals for bravery and doing research in to the diet of soldiers. During the 1930s he researched the benefits of milk in the diets of mothers, children and the poor. He went on to study the problems of nutrition in many areas of the world. In 1936 he published a report called Food, Health and Income. *It showed that the cost of a basic nutritious diet was too expensive for half the British population and that 10% of the population were undernourished. His report became the basis for the British Government's food and rationing policy during World War Two.*

▲ **SOURCE G** Extract from the Official Website of the Nobel Foundation. The scientific study into the goodness of food people eat was new in the twentieth century. The Scotsman, John Boyd-Orr was one of the first people to carry out such a study.

enquiry

How were the first chemical cures for diseases and infections discovered?

☑ **EXAM TIP**

Use the information in this book to make a timeline showing when the causes of different diseases were discovered and who discovered them. You should learn these and use them to support your answers to exam questions with detailed examples.

In the early twentieth century, based on the work of Pasteur and Koch, the search for chemical drugs to fight disease got underway. Paul Ehrlich called these chemicals 'magic bullets' because they killed only the germ that caused a particular disease.

The following individuals each made an important contribution to the discovery of cures for diseases:

Paul Ehrlich *(1854–1915)*

Ehrlich became a doctor of medicine in 1878 in Germany. His main interest was in using chemical dyes to stain animal tissues so that they could be studied more easily under a microscope. In 1890 he went to work for Koch at the Institute for Infectious Diseases in Berlin. In 1896 he became the director of a new medical research institute at Steglitz in Berlin where he worked with Emil von Behring on a serum to prevent diphtheria.

At this time the germ that causes syphilis was discovered. Ehrlich decided to try and find a chemical that would destroy this germ. After testing with hundreds of drugs his team failed to find the cure. Dr Sahachiro Hata, had succeeded in infecting rabbits with the germ and Ehrlich asked him to re-test some of the chemical drugs on the infected rabbits. He found that the 606th drug worked. The first magic bullet had been discovered. He called it 'Salvarsan 606'. The year was 1908.

Gerhard Domagk *(1895–1964)*

Domagk went to work for I G Farben, a German chemical company in 1927. He tested thousands of chemicals, on animals, for their magic bullet properties. In 1932 he tested a red dye called Prontosil, but all the animals he tested it on died. Later Domagk discovered that if he added other substances to the dye it could slow down or stop infections in mice caused by the streptococcal bacteria. In 1935 he was about to publish his findings when his daughter, Hildegard, pricked her finger with a needle. She became infected with the streptococcal bacteria and was close to death. Her father injected her with Prontosil and she made a complete recovery. This second magic bullet was one of a group of drugs known as sulphonamides and was far more powerful than Salvarsan 606. It was found to stop many infections such as pneumonia and meningitis. Domagk won the Nobel Prize in 1939, but Hitler did not wish Germans to contaminate themselves with foreign awards and instead stamped the Sulphonomide patent with the Nazi swastika.

QUESTION

How important was the work of individuals like Ehrlich, Domagk and Fleming in curing diseases and infections in the early twentieth century? Support your answer with reasons and examples. When writing your answer think of what each person did and the factors that helped them such as:

- war

- chance

- science and technology

- individual initiative.

Now decide which of these things was the most important in finding cures for diseases and infections.

Concluding your enquiry:

How were the first chemical cures for diseases and infections discovered?

You should be able to make a timeline showing when the chemical cures were discovered and who discovered them. Use this to add detailed examples to your answer.

Alexander Fleming
(1881–1955)

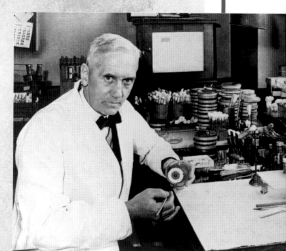

Fleming moved to London when he was 14. His father had died and he went to live with his brother who had a medical practice in the city. After working for a shipping firm and volunteering for the Boer War he was encouraged by his brother to enter the medical profession. He got top marks in his examinations and could have worked anywhere. He chose St Mary's Hospital in London because he had once played water polo against them! In 1905 he switched from surgery to bacteriology so that he could stay in the rifle club at St Mary's. In 1909 Ehrlich visited London and Fleming became one of the few doctors to use salvarsan. He gained a reputation for treating many well-known London people for syphilis. He was so successful that he gained the nickname 'Private 606' after the number that Paul Ehrlich had given to the first magic bullet.

During the First World War Fleming worked with his colleagues in a battlefield hospital laboratory in France. He made many improvements to the treatment of the wounded. He was convinced that deaths would have been avoided if a chemical could be found to fight simple infections caused by germs getting into the soldiers' wounds.

In the 1920s he went back to his laboratory in London to study nose drops and tears that seemed to kill weaker infections. In 1928, in his untidy laboratory, he made an accidental discovery. While tidying up he noticed a mysterious mould growing in one of his petri dishes that seemed to have killed all the harmful staphylococci bacteria around it. He examined the mould and found it was penicillin. The properties of penicillin had been known about for over one hundred years. Fleming wrote up and published his findings in 1929. He continued to study the mould but concluded that as it lost its properties when mixed with blood in test tubes, it would not work on living tissue. Fleming failed to do the obvious experiment with laboratory animals to see if penicillin could cure infection in living tissue.

It took another 10 years before the potential of penicillin to destroy many harmful bacteria was fully realised.

The discovery of

Historians, including the Canadian scientist Jules Brunel, have shown that Alexander Fleming's discovery that penicillin mould kills bacteria had been published earlier by others, notably Bartolomeo Gosio of Rome in 1896, and E. Duchesnes of Lyons in 1897.

◀ **SOURCE A** From *History of Medicine. A Scandalously Short Introduction* by Jacalyn Duffin, 2000.

The Role of Howard Florey

The summer of 1940 awoke the dreaming spires (of Oxford) with air-raid sirens. The war was beginning to bite.

In an annex of the Oxford medical school's Pathology Department a construction of inverted lemonade bottles, bedpans, rubber tubes, glass pipes, a mahogany bookshelf from the Bodleian (library), a milk churn, bathtub, bronze letter box and electric bell was manufacturing the most necessary drug of the century.

The Professor of Pathology was Howard Walter Florey (1898–1968), an Australian from Adelaide. He had arrived in Oxford from being Professor of Pathology in Sheffield in 1935 and like many an academic new broom swept his young assistants into the Science Library to find neglected or abandoned research worth reviving.

It struck Florey that some work reported by Professor Alexander Fleming in 1929 might be worth an experiment. His German-Russian chemist Ernst Chain grew the mould in brewer's yeast and extracted its juice. On 12th February 1941 Florey tried it in the Radcliffe Infirmary, on a policeman with staphylococcal septicaemia following a scratch on the mouth whilst pruning his rose bushes. So little penicillin had been produced that they had to bicycle his urine up the road to the Pathology Department for the remains of the penicillin to be extracted and reused. The patient showed a definite improvement. The clinical trial was a success. Sadly the penicillin ran out and the patient died.

▲ **SOURCE B** From *The Alarming History of Medicine* by Richard Gordon, 1993.

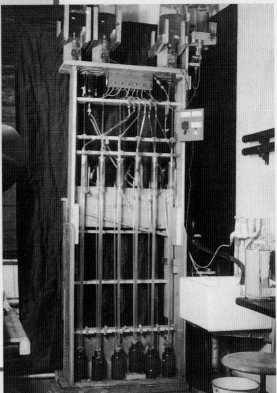

▲ **SOURCE C** The world's first penicillin factory in the Sir William Dunn School of Pathology, Oxford University.

penicillin

The Role of Ernst Chain

Ernst Chain (1906–79) had studied biochemistry, and had continued research in the field until Adolf Hitler became Chancellor (of Germany) in 1933. Though born in Berlin and a naturalized citizen, Chain realised that as a part-Russian Jew with leftward political leanings, he may have better opportunities elsewhere. He left for Great Britain almost as soon as Hitler took power. Unfortunately, in the years that followed he could not get his mother or sister out of the country. His mother died in a concentration camp and his sister disappeared.

It was Chain who uncovered Alexander Fleming's paper on penicillin as part of his larger research into antibiotics, together with Howard Florey. They found that penicillin in fact was not an enzyme, and Chain worked out its structure.

◀ **SOURCE D** A Science Odyessy: People and Discoveries: Ernst Chain.

The problems of mass production

The potential of using penicillin to treat wounded soldiers was immediately recognised in the Second World War (1939–45). However the concept of antibiotics was new, and a practical method for large-scale production was not available. Treatments required from one to two million Oxford units of the substance. The urgency of finding a method for mass-producing penicillin led to international co-operation. In the United States, the task was assigned to Andrew J. Moyer (1899–1959) who found that by culturing penicillin mould in a culture broth comprising corn steep liquor and lactose, penicillin yields could be greatly increased. These discoveries led to industrial penicillin production, which saved thousands of lives during the war.

▲ **SOURCE E** From the National Inventors Hall of Fame website.

Fleming, Florey and Chain were jointly awarded the Nobel Prize for the discovery of penicillin in 1945.

QUESTIONS

1 Read Source A and the information on Alexander Fleming on page 143. Source A says that knowledge of the anti-bacterial properties of penicillin had been published well before Fleming published his findings in 1929. Explain why many history books give Fleming the credit for discovering penicillin.

2 Read Source B and study Source C. What contribution did Florey and Chain make in the development of penicillin as a medicine?

3 Read Sources D and E. War was the most important factor in the development of penicillin as the first antibiotic drug. Do you agree with this interpretation?

Use the sources and your knowledge to help you to explain your answer.

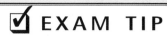

☑ EXAM TIP

When you are asked how important a factor like the work of an individual is in the development of medicine, always compare its importance with other factors like war, science, chance and government action.

enquiry

What impact did the two World Wars have on medicine in the modern world?

It is estimated that about 20 million people died because of military action in the First World War (1914–18), and another 30 million in the Second World War (1939–1945). These figures do not include the huge number of people who were injured.

Doctors and surgeons in many fields of medicine gave their services to help relieve the sufferings caused by war and the evidence shows that many improvements were made as a result. Many of these developments relied on the research and discoveries made in the nineteenth century.

What medical changes took place during the First World War (1914–18)?

The Armed Forces

Interest in the health of the population in general and the armed forces in particular grew as a result of war.

> *The general health of the Grand Fleet has been extremely good, indeed, probably better than in times of peace. The average daily percentage of sick in the whole Fleet in 1913 was 2.37%, and in 1914 a little lower, 2.03%. Since the outbreak of war daily sickness in the Grand Fleet has been almost always under 1%. Most of the sickness was of a minor character, such as seasonal influenza and boils.*

▲ **SOURCE A** Statement by General H D Rolleston, RN, Consultant Physician to the Royal Navy, to the London Medical Society on 12th February 1917.

The health of Britain's sailors began to improve and this was put down to the following factors:

- Comparative isolation of the fleets leading to less drunkenness and sexually transmitted diseases.

- Quarantine restrictions in drafting men from shore (they were kept in barracks to be checked for diseases before being allowed back onto the ships).

- Lectures on personal hygiene.

- Measures to remove the effects of boredom such as competitions and cinema films.

- Improvement in the ventilation of ships.

Life-saving technology

William Rontgen had discovered X-rays in 1895 and, soon after, hospitals began to use them to look for disease and broken bones inside the body, but it was during the First World War that they became really important. Mobile X-ray machines were used on the battlefront in France and Belgium so that soldiers with bullet and shrapnel wounds could be treated more quickly and effectively.

Marie Curie realised that X-rays could save soldiers' lives so she temporarily gave up her work at the Radium Institute in Paris and convinced the French government to set up the Red Cross Radiology Service. By October 1914 she had the first of 20 radiology vehicles. These X-ray vans transported the essential equipment to the battlefront and were known by the soldiers as '*Petites Curies*' (little Curies).

Blood transfusions had been tried ever since William Harvey had discovered the circulation of blood. They were unsuccessful in most cases but no one knew why until Landsteiner discovered blood groups in 1900. Even then it was not possible to store blood because it clotted so quickly. War injuries led to many men dying from loss of blood and surgical shock. A solution to the problems of storing blood was needed. In 1914 it was discovered that sodium citrate stopped blood from clotting, and during the First World War American army doctor, O.H. Robertson, used this method to keep blood fresh so that it could be used to help British soldiers. In the 1940s he showed that mixing this blood with a natural sugar would allow the blood to be stored for up to three weeks.

Plastic Surgery

The flood of casualties from the Battle of the Somme and the dedication of Harold Gillies, a British Army surgeon, led to the development of Queen's Hospital in Kent as the major centre for facial and plastic surgery. It was opened in 1917 and provided over 1000 beds. Over 5000 servicemen were admitted in the years between 1917 and 1921.

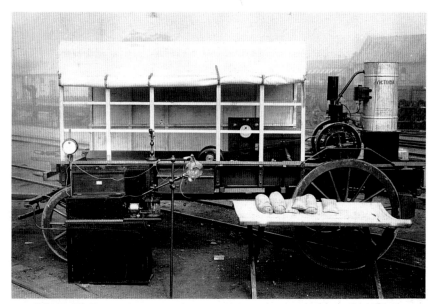

▲ **SOURCE B** A Petite Curie.

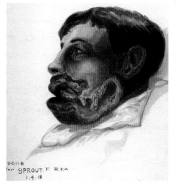
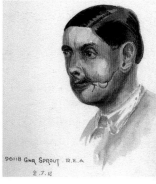

▲ **SOURCE C** Gunner Sprout was one of the soldiers treated at Queen's Hospital. The pictures show him before and after surgery.

☑ EXAM TIP

This is a difficult question to answer and would carry 12 marks, so leave time to plan your answer. Do not spend too much time on questions that carry fewer marks, and therefore, require shorter answers.

QUESTION

The First World War only speeded up developments in medicine that would have happened anyway as a result of discoveries in the nineteenth century. Do you agree?

Use the information on these pages and in earlier sections of the book to explain your answer.

Plan your answer:

Think about how the First World War speeded up developments in:

- health education
- medical technology for diagnosis
- improvements in surgery.

Did these developments depend on discoveries in the nineteenth century? Give examples. Would these developments have happened if there had not been a First World War? Now say whether or not you agree or disagree and why.

enquiry

How did Sir Archibald McIndoe contribute to improvements in medicine during the Second World War (1939–1945)?

Archibald McIndoe (1900–1960) was born on the 4th May, 1900, in Dunedin, New Zealand. His father was a printer and Archibald was the second of four children. He qualified as a doctor in 1924, winning medals in medicine and surgery, but went to work at the Mayo Clinic in the United States as an anatomist in 1925. His work resulted in the publication of several medical papers. An English Lord, living in the USA at the time, was so impressed with his surgical skill that he encouraged him to look for a position in England.

McIndoe arrived in London in the winter of 1930 only to find that there was no suitable appointment for him. His cousin was Sir Harold Gillies (see page 147) and he suggested an appointment as clinical assistant in the Department of Plastic Surgery at St Bartholomew's Hospital. From here McIndoe went on to an exceptional career in plastic surgery working at many famous London hospitals. He was a natural artist, very determined, quick at making decisions and extremely hard working.

In 1938, McIndoe was appointed Consultant in Plastic Surgery to the Royal Air Force. At the outbreak of war in 1939, he chose the Queen Victoria Hospital at East Grinstead because he considered it a suitable site for setting up a centre for plastic and jaw surgery. This was the start of the Battle of Britain and the hospital was close to the major RAF fighter airfields. He always refused to join the armed services because this would have meant that he would have been under government control like a civil servant.

McIndoe's work in rehabilitating badly burned aircrew, not only physically but also psychologically, was quite outstanding. Richard Hillary, a terribly burned fighter pilot who was later killed in action gives a graphic account in his book *The Last Enemy* of what he and others like him owe to McIndoe. McIndoe fought to improve the pay and conditions of 'his boys'. He even lent them money to set them up in civilian life. The 'Guinea Pig Club' preserves his memory by an annual meeting at East Grinstead attended by members from all over the world.

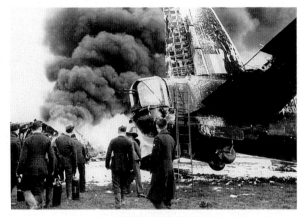

▲ **SOURCE A** Flames encircle a Vickers Wellington bomber during the Second World War. Between 1940 and 1945, 3,600 rescued aircrew sustained burns to the hands and face.

> ☑ **EXAM TIP**
>
> When answering questions which ask for reasons, try to pick out the most important and explain your choice. Do not simply list your reasons.

QUESTIONS

1 Suggest reasons why the fighter pilots who were treated by McIndoe called themselves 'The Guinea Pig Club'.

2 'McIndoe's brilliant career was no accident but due to a combination of factors.' Do you agree with this comment? Use your knowledge to explain your answer.

Why did the British Government's attitude towards health care change at the end of the Second World War?

By the end of the Second World War one of the great obstacles to successful surgery had been solved with the mass production of penicillin (see page 145). The real impact of this war on health in Britain was, however, much greater than a simple series of individual discoveries. A combination of important events and the work of individuals had caused major changes in the attitude of the government that led to a revolution in health care over the ten years from 1939 to 1949:

- The work of Sir William Beveridge and Aneurin Bevan.

- The experience of the First World War and the Great Depression of the 1930s.

- Changes in politics.

- The need to rebuild Britain after the destruction of the Second World War.

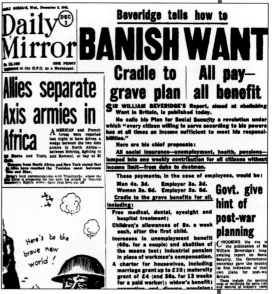

▲ **SOURCE B** The front page from the *Daily Mirror*, 2nd December, 1942.

How did individuals help to bring about changes to health services in Britain between 1939 and 1949?

William Beveridge *(1879–1963)*

Beveridge was the son of a judge. He went to Oxford University and was trained in the law. When Lloyd George introduced Labour Exchanges and unemployment insurance in 1911, Beveridge was given the job of organising the national system. He used his great knowledge of social insurance schemes from 1911 to 1939 to produce the Beveridge Report of 1942. The report argued for a comprehensive scheme of health and social insurance for everyone, not just employed workers as in 1911. He became a Liberal MP in 1944. The Labour government, elected in 1945, was able to use his ideas to support their case for a National Health Service.

Aneurin Bevan *(1897–1960)*

Bevan was the son of a Welsh coal miner who went down the pit himself at the age of 13. He overcame a severe stammer to become the chairman of his local branch of the South Wales Miners' Federation. In 1929 he was elected Labour MP for Ebbw Vale. As Minister of Health for the Labour government in 1946 he introduced the Bill for a national health service with these words: *Medical treatment should be made available to rich and poor alike in accordance with medical need and no other criteria. Worry about money in a time of sickness is a serious hindrance to recovery, apart from its unnecessary cruelty.*

enquiry

How did the experiences of the First World War and the Great Depression of the 1930s lead to changes in attitudes to public health in Britain?

Poverty and poor health were still features of life for many people during the 1920s and 1930s. Governments after 1918 had failed to produce 'a fit country for heroes to live in' promised by Lloyd George after the First World War. A visit to the doctor had to be paid for and not all families could afford treatment.

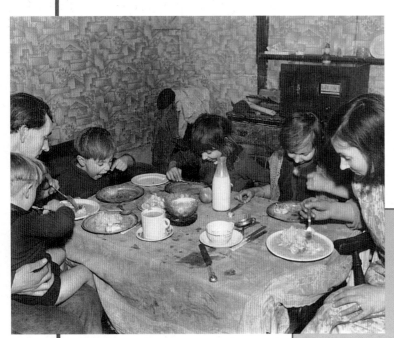

▲ **SOURCE A** Alfred Smith and his family at home in January 1939. Alfred Smith was an unemployed Londoner and his story appeared in the magazine Picture Post on 21st January 1939.

Mrs Evans' Story, 1938

In the middle of February I went down with the flu. I was poorly for a fortnight and couldn't get out of bed. I had to rely on Alec my husband, and my two children, John and Elsie, to run the house. John and Alec then got flu. Alec was worried about having time off work, so he carried on going to the factory. John went into school because he didn't want to miss his lessons – he was studying for a place at the grammar school. After a couple of days it was obvious they were getting worse – they had high temperatures, were sick and started to complain about pains in their chests. I was so worried that I got them up and went round to the doctor's house. We went into the doctor's kitchen and he sat John on the kitchen table and listened to his chest. Then he examined Alec and said it was pneumonia, and that they both needed hospital care. We took Alec into the hospital straight away – as a workingman his treatment was covered by National Health Insurance. I made the doctor tell me how to look after John as we couldn't afford hospital treatment for him – I really wished we'd paid into the hospital scheme, but 3d a week (1.25p) seemed so much when we're so rarely ill.

QUESTION

How useful are Sources A and B to an historian researching health and living conditions in the early twentieth century?

▲ **SOURCE B** This was the experience of a family with an employed father. Think how much worse it must have been for the millions of families unemployed because of the Great Depression that was affecting Britain and the world in the 1930s. In 1932 it was estimated that 2.5 million people in Britain were unemployed.

How did changes in politics affect attitudes to public health in the 1920s and 1930s?

In 1918 all men over 21 and women over 30 had been given the vote. Liberal politicians supported by a small but growing Labour Party had forced through health and housing reforms (see Source D on page 140) but the problems of the 1930s and the huge government debts caused by depression and the First World War meant, that for the time being, a National Health Service was out of the question. Some people believed it was wrong in principle for the government to provide free health care.

> *I am unable to accept the proposal to set up a national medical service based upon the family doctor. The dangerous habit of getting something for nothing will be encouraged which is bound to have a damaging effect on the morale of the people.*

▲ **SOURCE C** Sir Andrew Grierson, in 'Report of the Committee on a Scottish Health Service', 1936.

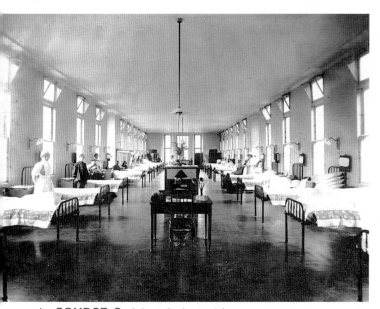

▲ **SOURCE C** A hospital ward in the early twentieth century. Before the National Health Service was created in 1948 hospitals treated mainly poor people as the rich had their treatment at home or in nursing homes.

How did the Second World War lead to the creation of the National Health Service?

As well as hardship and terror, the war also brought some benefits such as better health and higher earnings. Average weekly earnings rose by 80% between 1938 and 1945. Thanks mainly to rationing and government food subsidies the cost of living rose by less than half of this and unemployment largely disappeared. Many people were now employed in the armed forces or in making weapons. Far-reaching proposals were put forward to improve the future of those who had been called upon to make sacrifices in the war. When the Labour government was elected in 1945 it promised to introduce a National Health Service as soon as possible. This service would be free and available to everyone, in the phrase they used at the time, 'from the Cradle to the Grave'.

Concluding your enquiry:
What impact did the two world wars have on medicine in the modern world? Divide your answer into two:

- medical developments
- public health developments in Britain.

For each part of your answer describe the work of the key individuals and how war influenced what they did.

enquiry

What has happened to the National Health Service since 1948?

The National Health Service Act was passed in 1946 but there was much opposition from people who felt that the government would now be interfering far too much in people's lives. Many also believed that the service would be far too expensive and would lead to higher and higher taxes. The main opposition came from the doctors themselves. Many felt that they would be paid less if they could not charge patients and that the government would end up telling them how to treat their patients.

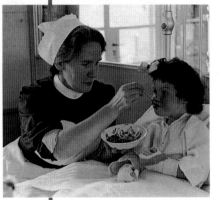

▲ **SOURCE A** A nurse treating a child in hospital in the 1950s.

Despite all the opposition, Bevan (see page 149) won the argument in Parliament and on 5th July 1948 the National Health Service began offering free treatment and services for all including:

- Hospitals
- Eye tests and spectacles
- Dental treatment and false teeth
- Visits to the local doctor (GP)
- Prescription medicine from the chemist
- Maternity and child welfare
- Ambulance and emergency service
- Vaccination programme
- Government controlled training of doctors and nurses
- Government controlled medical research.

Queues formed outside surgeries and hospitals as people tried to take advantage of the free service.

Dentists were booked solid for months in advance and the production of spectacles trebled in two years.

Why did the government introduce charges for some services?

The cost of the NHS doubled in the first two years. In 1950, the money ran out. The first charges for NHS services were introduced in that year with a 50% contribution towards false teeth and spectacles. Its founders had hoped that the cost of the NHS would actually fall within ten years as the benefits of better health care took effect. People who do not become ill do not need to use the Health Service. In fact the budget has risen ever since and charges for prescriptions, dental and other health services have been introduced.

How has the National Health Service changed since the late 1950s?

In the second half of the twentieth century the NHS became a victim of its own success. New technology, such as transplant surgery, was being introduced so quickly and more people were being treated using more expensive drugs and equipment. This led to an increase in the number of people wanting treatment and also meant that people would live longer and would then need care in the future. By 1987 waiting lists for medical treatment were growing and health authorities were in debt, causing many hospital wards to close. Patients who could afford to were paying for treatment so that they did not have to wait in NHS queues. This went against the principles declared in Bevan's speech of 1946, in which he introduced the National Health Service (see page 149).

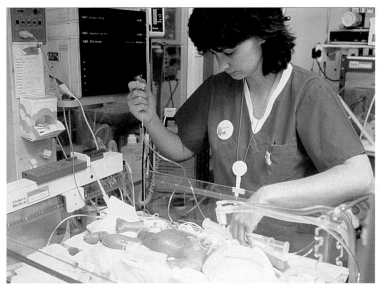

▲ SOURCE B A nurse caring for a newly born baby in a modern hospital maternity ward.

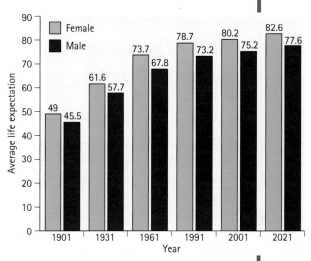

▲ SOURCE D Male and female life expectation in the United Kingdom.

QUESTION

In Source C Tony Blair said that 'the NHS was failing'. Source D shows that life expectancy is increasing. Is Source C a reliable source for historians investigating the NHS in the 1990s? Explain your answer.

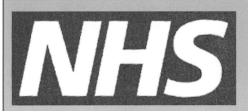

Foreword by the Prime Minister
Creating the NHS was the greatest act of modernisation ever achieved by Labour Government. It banished the fear of becoming ill that had for years blighted the lives of millions of people. But I know that one of the main reasons people elected a new Government on May 1st was their concern that the NHS was failing them and their families. In my contract with the people of Britain I promised that we would rebuild the NHS. We have already made a start. The Government is putting an extra £1.5 billion into the health service during the course of this year and next. More money is going into improving breast cancer and children's services. And new hospitals are being built. The NHS will get better every year so that it once again delivers dependable, high quality care - based on need, not ability to pay.
Tony Blair, 1997

▲ SOURCE C An extract from a speech about the NHS made by the Prime Minister, Tony Blair, in 1997.

Concluding your enquiry:
What has happened to the NHS since 1948? Make a list of the ways it has been improved. Make a list of the ways it has suffered problems.
Which list do you think is more important? Explain your answer.

enquiry

Did science and technology help or hinder medical progress in the twentieth century?

1903 Willem Einthoven invented the electrocardiograph to monitor the heart

1908 First successful transfusion using Landsteiner's blood types

1911 Marie Curie discovered radium later used in the treatment of cancer

1914 W H Howell was the first scientist to study blood using a microscope with ultraviolet light

1929 An artificial heart made of two bellows inside a brass container was developed at a Canadian university

1931 German scientists developed the electron microscope, which made it possible to see molecules

1935 First successful use of a heart-lung machine to keep an animal alive

1937 First blood bank set up in Chicago. Refrigerated blood lasted ten days

1944 Surgical repair of the heart in a living human performed in Stockholm

1951 Dr Clarence Dennis performed the first open heart surgery but the patient died

1957 A doctor and an electronics engineer developed the first portable pacemaker to keep the heartbeat steady

1958 Two American doctors began experiments in animal heart transplants

1967 Dr Christian Barnard performed the first successful human heart transplant in South Africa

1984 A baby's heart was replaced with a baboon's heart

Is the surgeon more important than the scientist in a modern hospital?

Before the twentieth century instruments like the thermometer and the stethoscope had been invented. These allowed doctors to measure and hear problems in the body but only if the patient came to them with an illness. Even then they could only examine internal problems if the body was opened up and this remained a risky business because of the danger of infection.

X-ray technology or radiography solved this problem. A series of discoveries and technical developments made it possible to see inside the chest and brain and identify problems which the patient may not yet be aware of. This could now be done as a matter of routine without the need for risky surgery. The doctor could now decide whether or not the patient was ill.

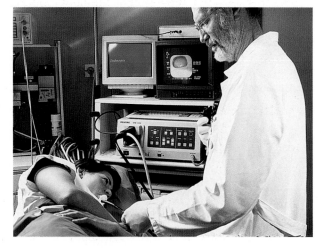

▶ **SOURCE A**
Doctor about to perform an endoscopy examination of a patient's stomach. The technique involves inserting a flexible fibre-optic viewing tube into the oesophagus. A light at the end of the tube illuminates the body and the view is shown on the monitor.

How has technology changed our hospitals?

This new technology in medicine brought great changes in the late twentieth century. Hospitals became places for scientific investigation and cure. They were full of expensive equipment. The very sick needed the life support that could only be provided in hospitals. Those who were not critically ill came to hospital for diagnosis, which also required expensive machinery.

The chronically ill, the homeless and the disabled – the very people who used to be in hospital – were less welcome. The expensive treatment using modern technology led to financial crisis in the health services of many countries in the 1990s resulting in the closure of hospital wards and long waits for operations (see pages 152–153).

What made successful organ transplants possible?

Skin and eyes were among the first successful transplants, but transplanting larger internal organs like the heart posed countless problems. The kidney was the first such organ to be successfully transplanted.

In Britain, Peter Medawar had been researching the topic of transplant rejection, which he had observed in skin grafts as a wartime surgeon. He found that the grafts often failed because the body's immune system developed antibodies to fight against the skin graft because it did not belong to that body.

In 1954, at a hospital in the USA, Richard Herrick lay dying from kidney disease. His identical twin brother Ronald donated one of his kidneys and it was successfully transplanted into his brother. Because they were identical twins, the organ did not appear foreign to Richard's body, and so it was not rejected.

Further research showed that the body could be bombarded with X-rays to destroy the immune system, which prevented rejection, but this amount of radiation often killed the patient. In 1959 doctors discovered the drug imuran, which stopped the body rejecting organs without killing the patient and, in 1960, discovered tissue typing which, like blood typing discovered in 1900, matched the transplant organ to the patient. The transplant breakthrough had been made and between 1954 and 1973 about 10,000 kidney transplants were performed.

Today the main problem for transplant surgery is that there are far more patients waiting for transplant organs than there are organs available. According to the Novartis Pharmaceuticals Corporation of America, in 1996 there were 2,340 heart, 805 lung, 39 heart-lung and 4,000 liver transplants performed in the USA, but in 1997 there were 3,900 patients waiting for a heart transplant, 2,700 for a lung, 235 for a heart-lung and 9,600 for a liver.

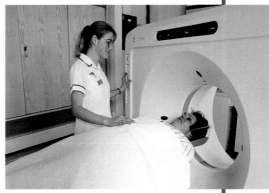

▲ SOURCE B A patient in a scanner.

QUESTION

Write down five ways in which science and technology have caused problems in medicine since 1900.

Which of the following factors has caused most change in surgery since 1900?

- Scientific discoveries

- Technological developments

- War

- Government action

- The work of individuals

You will need to refer back to earlier enquiries to help you to answer the last part of this enquiry.

Concluding your enquiry:
Did science and technology help or hinder medical progress in the twentieth century?
Write down five ways in which science and technology have improved medicine since 1900.

☑ **EXAM TIP**

Use this enquiry to make sure you understand the difference between science and technology as factors in the development of medicine over time.

enquiry

> What are the main dangers to human health in the modern world?

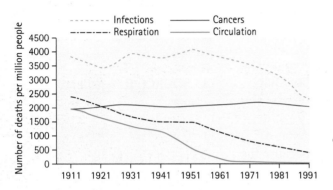

▲ **SOURCE A** The main causes of death, and the numbers of people who die from them in the UK.

☑ EXAM TIP

When you are asked questions about a modern world topic, try to use specific and detailed examples from your own knowledge of modern events to support your answer. Remember that textbooks are always out of date.

How have 'old' diseases increased?

- **Mumps** (infectious disease marked by swelling of the glands on the neck)
  In 1999 there were 358 cases of this once common childhood disease but that figure rose in 2000 to 654. The Public Health Laboratory Service has put this down to young people who were too old to be given the MMR vaccine first introduced in 1988 for measles, mumps and rubella.

- **Asthma** (illness causing difficulty in breathing)
  The National Asthma Campaign estimates that, in the year 2000, one in every seven children and one in every 25 adults was affected by asthma. Research in Leicester showed that the number of cases in under-fives almost doubled between 1990 and 1998.

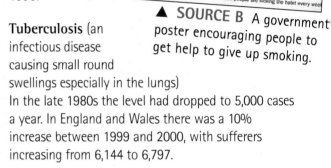

▲ **SOURCE B** A government poster encouraging people to get help to give up smoking.

- **Tuberculosis** (an infectious disease causing small round swellings especially in the lungs)
  In the late 1980s the level had dropped to 5,000 cases a year. In England and Wales there was a 10% increase between 1999 and 2000, with sufferers increasing from 6,144 to 6,797.

- **Malaria** (an infectious disease caused by the bite of some mosquitoes)
  The last truly British epidemic of this disease was recorded in Rochester, Kent, in 1918 when many First World War soldiers came home from Greece with the mosquito-transmitted disease. After the war the numbers infected continued to fall until the 1950s when the numbers of people travelling abroad shot up again. Today there are about 2,000 cases a year brought in from abroad.

- **Eczema**
  This unpleasant skin complaint is on the increase. In the 1970s about 9% of children were affected but by 1999 that figure had risen to about 20%.

- **Diabetes** (an illness in which the body has problems controlling its sugar levels)
  Experts believe that about 2.4 million people suffered from this illness in 2001. More than a million children under 16 were classed as overweight or obese in the year 2000. Doctors are reported to be convinced that junk food and a lack of exercise is causing many children to contract traditionally middle-aged diseases such as diabetes.

Is prevention of disease better than cure?

Many of the conditions mentioned are unpleasant but not a threat to life or long-term health in people who are otherwise fit. The fact that modern medicine does not seem to be able wipe them out altogether has led some health experts to look towards prevention rather than cure.

Can your lifestyle permanently damage your health?

HOW EUROPE COMPARES

Percentage of 15-to 16-year-olds who have used any type of illicit drugs in their lifetime (1999)		Percentage of 15- and 16-year-olds who reported daily smoking at the age of 13 or younger (1999)		Percentage of 15-16-year-olds who have been drunk 20 times or more in a lifetime (1999)	
UK	36	UK	20	Denmark	41
Ireland	32	Ireland	18	UK	29
Italy	26	Moscow	16	Ireland	25
Denmark	25	Finland	15	Finland	28
Poland	18	France	14	Sweden	19
Iceland	16	Denmark	12	Norway	16
Norway	13	Norway	11	Poland	11
Portugal	12	Sweden	10	Moscow	10
Finland	10	Portugal	8	France	4
Sweden	9	Italy	6	Greece	4
Malta	8	Cyprus	5	Portugal	4
Cyprus	3	Greece	3	Cyprus	2

▲ **SOURCE C** From a survey by the Alcohol and Health Research Centre in Edinburgh, reported in *The Independent* Wednesday, 21st February 2001.

QUESTION

Why might the figures in the survey by the Alcohol and Health Research Centre, be unreliable?

Does modern food make you ill?

In the early 1980s Health Minister Edwina Currie caused an outcry when she suggested that most of the eggs we ate contained the salmonella virus, which can cause food poisoning. In the late 1980s BSE was found in British cattle and quickly spread to Europe. The Southwood Report of 1989 stated that it was 'most unlikely that BSE would have any effects on human health'. Government ministers tried to persuade the public that it was safe to eat beef. In 1996 a new type of CJD had been identified in young people. The most likely explanation for this was that their illness was linked to eating beef from cattle with BSE.

Such incidents have made people much more careful about the food they eat. Some have turned to vegetarianism, others have demanded that animals be fed organically and that crops are grown organically. Government regulation of the food industry has increased accordingly.

KEY WORDS

CJD – Creutzfeldt-Jacob Disease, which is a rare and fatal brain disease

BSE – Bovine Spongiform Encephalopathy or 'mad cow disease'

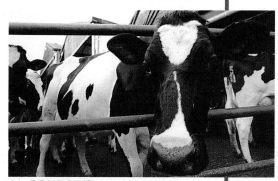

▲ **SOURCE D** From the *Daily Mail*, Monday 26th March 2001. The caption for the photo read, 'Do you want meat and milk from healthy cattle or drug-induced freaks with terrible illnesses?'

Concluding your enquiry:

What are the main dangers to human health in the modern world?

Keep a diary of 'health-scare stories' from the newspapers and TV news as they happen over the next two weeks. In these stories, which of the following are shown to be the biggest causes of ill-health in the modern world?

- life style, or
- poor food hygiene, or
- inadequate medical care, or
- poverty.

Explain your answer with examples from your research.

enquiry

> ## What alternative treatments do people in the modern world use?

What is acupuncture?

Acupuncture points are believed to stimulate the central nervous system (the brain and spinal cord) to release natural chemicals into the muscles, spinal cord and brain. These chemicals either change the experience of pain or release other chemicals that influence the body's self-regulating systems. The biochemical changes may stimulate the body's natural healing abilities and promote physical and emotional well being.

Acupuncture is one of the oldest, most commonly used medical procedures in the world. It originated in China more than 2,000 years ago and became widely known in the United States in 1971 when *New York Times* reporter, James Reston, wrote about how doctors in Beijing, China, used needles to ease his pain after surgery. Research shows that acupuncture is helpful in treating a variety of health conditions.

In the past 20 years, acupuncture has grown in popularity in the United States. In 1993, the US Food and Drug Administration estimated that Americans made 9 to 12 million visits per year to acupuncture practitioners and spent as much as $500 million on acupuncture treatments. In 1995, an estimated 10,000 nationally certified acupuncturists were practising in the United States. By the year 2000, that number had doubled. An estimated one-third of certified acupuncturists in the United States are medical doctors.

Can a disease be cured by simply believing it is cured?

The term 'placebo' was long used in medicine for a prescribed substance thought to be medically inactive but helpful for controlling neurotic patients by giving them something which they believed would make them better. The word comes from the Latin 'I shall please'.

There are many unanswered questions but, by the late 1970s, it appeared as if both doctors and scientists had accepted the placebo effect as very important in medicine. It was seen as one of the body's methods of self-protection.

> *You cannot write a prescription without the element of the placebo.*
> *A prayer to Jupiter starts the prescription.*
> *It carries weight, the weight of two or three thousand years of medicine.*

▲ **SOURCE A** Eugene F Dubois, Professor of Medicine at Cornell University.

Are doctors and scientists always right?

In the mid-1960s, an apparently new illness, coronary heart disease, was suddenly discovered to be killing thousands of men prematurely. This disease, almost unknown in the mid-1920s, had increased very rapidly every year to become the commonest form of early death in males. The myth was launched that a high fat diet, resulting in cholesterol infiltrating the walls of the arteries to the heart, was the cause. Consequently, a low

> *Put bluntly, the facts have been selected and edited, preventing their proper interpretation, and it is not surprising that when we turn to the circumstantial evidence that is held to underpin the relationship between high-fat diet and heart disease, we find it has been similarly edited.*

▲ **SOURCE B** Dr Le Fanu in *Not Just Tobacco: Health Scares, Medical Paternalism and Individual Liberty*, by Chris R. Tame and David Botsford, 1996.

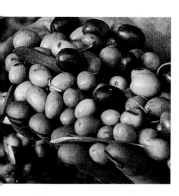

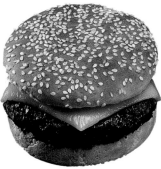

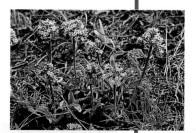

▶ **SOURCE C** Valerian is a herb used to make people sleep. Culpeper's book, *The Complete Herbal*, published in 1655, traces the use of this herb back to the Ancient Greeks.

fat diet was officially promoted as the 'new healthy diet'. Statistical evidence was presented in order to support this claim, however some doctors disagreed with this as shown in Source B.

While many still believe that simply reducing fat intake will lower the risk of heart disease, it has become apparent that the quality, not the quantity, of fat is the key to good health.

In 1972, heart disease expert Robert C Atkins, MD, created quite a stir when he published his first book, advocating a high-protein, high-fat, low-carbohydrate diet as the best way to slow down or reverse heart disease. At the very least, Atkin's diet has demonstrated that it is possible to lose weight and to normalise cholesterol and blood pressure while on a diet high in fat.

Are herbal remedies better than modern drugs?

In the year 2000, the findings of a clinical study of 128 subjects, from 1982, found that the herb valerian produced 'significant improvement in sleep quality' without the hang-over effects commonly experienced with modern chemical sleeping pills.

In the late twentieth century alternative medicine became increasingly popular partly because it was supported and publicised by rich and famous individuals.

QUESTION

Why does it seem that more and more people in the modern world are using alternative treatments rather than western scientific medicine to try and cure illness?

Think about:

- The bad side effects of some modern drugs.
- The failure of modern medicine to stop some cancers and diseases.
- The dangers and risks of modern surgery.
- The long history of using herbal remedies.
- The support of important people for alternative medical treatments.

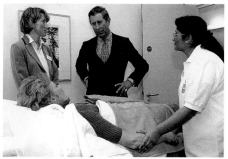

▲ **SOURCE D** The Prince of Wales speaking to a patient with breast cancer who is receiving aromatherapy treatment at the Haven Trust's support centre in London.

☑ EXAM TIP

Here is another way to answer 'why' question. Turn the five bullet points into a spider diagram and try to link them together. Now write a paragraph to explain what you have found.

Concluding your enquiry:

What alternative treatments do people in the modern world use?

Acupuncture and herbal remedies have been used for thousands of years. Can you think of reasons why they have become more popular as alternative methods of treatment only in the late twentieth century?

enquiry

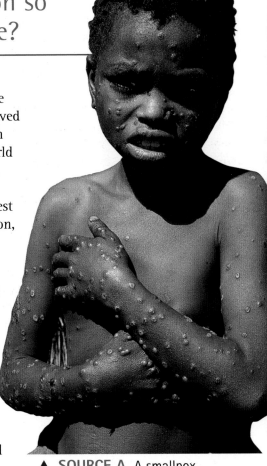

Why is the World Health Organisation so important in modern world medicine?

At the end of the Second World War the United Nations Conference on International Organisation in San Francisco unanimously approved a proposal by Brazil and China to set up a new international health organisation. The following year, 1946, the Constitution of the World Health Organisation (WHO) was approved in New York. On the 7th April, 1948, the 61 member states signed the constitution.

The objective of WHO is to help all peoples to reach the highest possible level of health. Health, as defined in the WHO constitution, is a state of complete physical, mental and social well-being and not merely the absence of disease and infirmity.

What has WHO done to improve health in the modern world?

In 1967, WHO began a campaign to eradicate smallpox. This was an enormous and complex exercise, which involved the vaccination of entire populations of countries in which smalllpox was prevalent. By 1972, the incidence of the disease had fallen rapidly. In 1980, the World Health Assembly declared that smallpox had been wiped out across the world.

Smallpox no longer affects anyone and the cost of getting rid of it – approximately $313 million over ten years – has been repaid many times in the saving of human lives and in the elimination of costs for vaccines, treatment and international surveillance activities.

▲ **SOURCE A** A smallpox sufferer in Africa before the disease was eradicated.

KEY WORDS

constitution –	a set of rules for an organisation like a government
endemic countries –	countries with a lot of cases of the disease
HIV –	Human Immunodeficiency Virus (this is the virus which will eventually cause AIDS)
AIDS –	Acquired Immune Deficiency Syndrome

Why is WHO spending so much time and money fighting against HIV/AIDS?

In 1987 the Global Programme on AIDS was launched within WHO. AIDS begins with HIV infection. As this develops in the infected person's body it gradually destroys immunity to other common infections and some forms of cancer, which eventually leads to illness and death. At the end of 2000 it was estimated that 36.1 million people worldwide were infected with most of them living in sub-Saharan Africa. According to the annual World Health Report AIDS had become the fourth biggest killer worldwide.

Where does HIV come from?

In trying to identify where AIDS originated there is a danger that people may try and use that debate to blame the disease on particular groups of individuals or certain lifestyles. The first cases of AIDS were reported in the USA in 1981 but research has shown that the disease may have started well before that. A plasma sample taken in 1959 from an adult male living in what is now the Democratic Republic of Congo was found to contain HIV infection. Other scientists have suggested that the infection could have existed even longer, perhaps around a hundred years or more ago.

It is now generally accepted that HIV/AIDS comes from SIV (Simian [monkey] Immunodeficiency Virus) carried by monkeys and chimpanzees. Researchers at Alabama University have suggested that HIV could have crossed over from chimpanzees as a result of a human killing a chimp and eating it for food. There are also other less likely theories:

- Polio vaccines used in the Congo in the 1950s were prepared using monkey kidneys. This may have transferred the virus to humans.

- HIV was manufactured by the CIA (US secret service) to use against its enemies.

- HIV was genetically engineered and brought out of the laboratory by accident.

Why has the AIDS epidemic spread so quickly since 1981?

Unprotected sex
There is some evidence that increasing numbers of young people are having sexual relations with more than one partner. When they do this without using condoms they stand a much greater chance of being infected by or infecting their partners.

International travel
'Patient Zero' was a Canadian flight attendant called Gaetan Dugas who travelled extensively worldwide. Several early cases of AIDS showed that the infected individuals were either direct or indirect sexual contacts of the flight attendant.

These cases could be traced to several different American cities showing how easily the infection could be spread around the world.

The blood industry
As blood transfusions became more and more common there was an increased demand for blood donors. In some cases the blood was not checked for HIV and some HIV infected blood was sent to countries all over the world.

Drug use
In the 1970s heroin became increasingly available following the Vietnam War. Addicts injected the drug into their blood stream and often shared needles. This meant that HIV could easily be passed on from one drug user to another through the blood left on the shared needle.

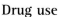

▲ SOURCE B
A cell infected with HIV.

QUESTION
What evidence can you find in this enquiry to argue that most health problems in the modern world are truly worldwide?

☑ EXAM TIP
You are asked to explain why the WHO is so important. You do not have to compare it to other organisations in such a question but you should try to explain the most important reason in your answer.

Concluding your enquiry:
Why is the World Health Organisation so important in modern world medicine?
Your answer to the Question will give you the best clue about what you need to write in order to conclude your enquiry.

enquiry

How has the understanding of genetics affected medicine?

1863 Gregor Mendel discovered that parents pass their traits on to their children in discrete units now known as genes

1940 Oswald Avery discovered that DNA transforms genes

1953 Francis Crick, James Watson and others discovered the double-helix structure of DNA

1966 The genetic code was cracked to show the relationship between genes and the proteins they help to create

1976 Knowledge of DNA was applied for the first time to a human illness

1984 The defective gene responsible for Huntingdon's disease was identified

1986 The Human Genome Project was established to try and decode the entire sequence of human DNA

2001 The complete sequence of human DNA was discovered and published

Watson, Crick, Wilkins and the discovery of the double helix

On 28th February 1953, Francis Crick (born in England, 1916) walked into the Eagle pub in Cambridge, England, and declared that he and his colleague James Watson (born in USA, 1928), 'had found the secret of life'. That morning, Watson and Crick had discovered the 'double-helix' structure of DNA and that it can 'unzip' to make copies of itself. This confirmed suspicions that DNA carries life's hereditary information. It was not until decades later, during the age of genetic engineering, that the incredible power unleashed that day became vivid.

The men were in some ways an odd pair. Crick had moved into physics from chemistry and biology, fascinated by the line 'between the living and the non-living'. Watson had studied ornithology, then gave up birds for viruses, and then changed his area of study again.

At a conference in Naples, Watson saw a ghostly image of a DNA molecule created by X-ray crystallography. DNA, he had heard, might be the stuff genes are made of. 'A potential key to the secret of life was impossible to push out of my mind,' he later wrote. 'It was certainly better to imagine myself becoming famous than growing into a stifled academic who had never risked a thought.'

The third contributor to the DNA discovery was Maurice Wilkins (born in New Zealand, 1916). He was a physicist who during the Second World War had worked on the development of the atomic bomb in the Manhattan Project, California. In 1946 he moved into biophysics research and later he began X-ray studies of DNA and sperm heads. His studies confirmed Watson and Crick's idea about the double helix structure of DNA.

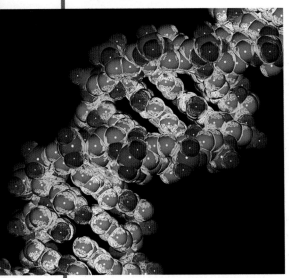

▲ **SOURCE A** The double helix structure of DNA as discovered by Watson, Crick and Wilkins.

KEY WORDS

DNA – Deoxyribonucleic Acid

proteins – any of a group of organic compounds that is essential for life

cancer – a disease resulting from a growth or tumour inside or outside the body

herpes – the name given to a group of inflammatory skin diseases including cold sores and shingles

Can genetics be used to cure people?

A cure for cancer?

The drug oltipraz was originally produced in the 1930s to fight infections. Now it seems it can provide a powerful boost to the body's natural anti-cancer defence systems. Professor David Lane, a cancer expert at Dundee University, has discovered how the 'cancer gene' P53 is a key factor in most instances of the disease. When it is damaged, cancer is more likely. Oltipraz seems to stop the poisons that damage P53.

Studies in China reportedly show that the drug clears poisons from the bodies of people who work in rice fields. These poisons are found in large amounts in mouldy rice and explain the high rate of liver cancer in that country.

Duncan's disease

The disease is named after the first family in whom the condition was recognised in 1975. An abnormal gene inherited only by boys causes it. Boys affected appear to be healthy and normal until they pick up a fairly common form of the **herpes** virus that infects the majority of people by adulthood. When they pick up the virus they become seriously ill and can die, sometimes very quickly.

Dr Bobby Gaspar, a clinical lecturer in immunology at Great Ormond Street Hospital, said that the discovery of the gene had made a vital difference in helping to diagnose the disease and in counselling families, and was opening the way for new treatments in the future.

Is gene testing safe?

An increasing number of gene tests are becoming available commercially. While some of these tests have greatly improved and even saved lives, scientists remain unsure about how to interpret many of them. Patients taking the tests face significant risks. If the tests show that they have a damaged gene that will cause them to die young or become seriously ill they may lose their job or be refused insurance. Because genetic information is shared, these risks can spread beyond them to their family members as well.

> *Cloning creates ordinary children who grow up to be unique. We are here to encourage scientific research and a good code of behaviour.*

▲ **SOURCE B** Severino Antinori, leader of a private international human cloning consortium.

> *Reproductive human cloning is not technically illegal in Britain, but the Human Fertilisation and Embryology Authority would certainly refuse permission. However, while some US states and countries, such as Japan, have banned it outright, others have not.*

▲ **SOURCE C** From *The Guardian*, Saturday, 10th March 2001.

QUESTIONS

1 Why do many people oppose the development of genetic medicine?

2 Is medical progress being made faster in the modern world than it has been in earlier times?

Use the information in this unit and your knowledge of progress in other periods of history to explain your answer.

Concluding your enquiry:

How has the understanding of genetics affected medicine?

You should consider how the understanding of genetics has both good and bad effects.

review

What progress has been made in improving health in the modern world?

The most important contribution to rising health standards in the twentieth century was the overall rise in living standards, and especially in diet, which reduced people's risk of dying from killer diseases like tuberculosis and typhus. Improvements in medical techniques in the early twentieth century made a much smaller contribution to rising health standards than is generally realised.

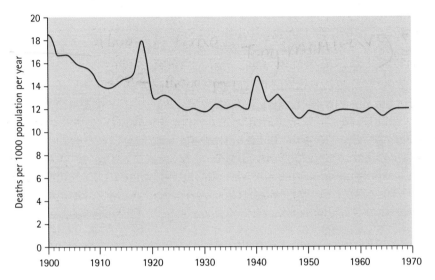

▲ **SOURCE A** Chart showing the death rate in the UK from 1900–1970 .

What problems have improvements in medicine and health in the modern world created?

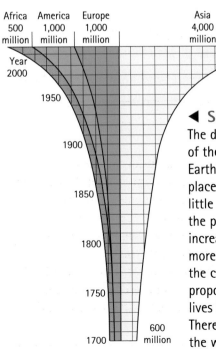

The benefits of modern medicine are very unevenly spread throughout the world. See pages 160–61 on the World Health Organisation.

◀ **SOURCE B** Population explosion: The diagram gives us a clear picture of the considerable expansion in the Earth's population that has taken place from the 1700s onwards. From little more than 600 million in 1700, the population of the world has increased to the 6300 million in 2000, more than half of which is found in the continent of Asia. A high proportion of the Earth's population lives in underdeveloped nations. Therefore the problems of caring for the world's population may increase.

> ☑ **EXAM TIP**
>
> Make sure you understand the importance of science and technology for developments in medicine in the modern world. Remember that they have not been the only factors in changing modern world medicine.

Is there any continuity in medicine in the modern world?

The short answer is that there is a lot of continuity because not all countries have been affected by the growth of science and technology in the same way as the West (Europe and the USA). Even in the West people still use old ideas. See pages 158–59 on alternative medicine.

We went to see a community of people that has grown up around a mganga (medicine man/witch doctor). He obviously does have some power (no matter if only psychological) over his patients. We saw him treat two women who were in a dead faint (or hypnotised we thought) with great ceremony and drum beating and yellow boiling liquid pumped into their ears. It was all a bit strange to us.

▲ **SOURCE C** An Englishman working in Tanzania (Africa) wrote this in a letter after visiting an isolated African village in February 1987.

Concluding your study of medicine:

In Question 2 on page 163 you were asked to compare medical progress in the modern world with medical progress in earlier times, such as:

- The nineteenth century when many improvements were being made in public health and surgery, and when Germ Theory was being developed.

- The Renaissance when there was great progress in the understanding of anatomy.

- The Ancient Roman period when progress was made in public health.

- The Ancient Greek period when natural treatments such as the Theory of the Four Humours and clinical observation were developed.

Your examination is about the history and development of medicine through time so it is very important for you to have an accurate chronological picture of what happened at different times. The best way to do this is to make your own time diagrams that show when important individuals lived and the factors that affected their lives and discoveries.

When you have made your diagrams you can put them in the correct order of time (chronology) to obtain a clear picture of how ideas from different periods might have affected each other, and when progress was fast or slow.

Glossary

Index